|| Hare Krishna ||

Animal Nutrition and Feed Technology

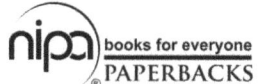

NIPA® GENX ELECTRONIC RESOURCES & SOLUTIONS P. LTD.
New Delhi-110 034

About the Author

Dr Raman Rao is presently a Professor of Animal Nutrition in the G.B. Pant University of Agriculture and Technology, Pantnagar [India]. He was awarded the **"Sir Stapledon's Commonwealth Fellowship" of England** to carryout Post - doctoral research at Dairy and Swine Research and Development Centre, Lennoxville (Québec), Canada. He had visited Boston (U.S.A.); Zürich, Interlaken, Jungfraujoch, Luzerne (Switzerland); Singen (Hohentwiel, Germany); Bon Accueil, Port Louis (Mauritius) and observed some cow barns, as being a patron - member of "International Society for Krishna Consciousness". He has been permitted by his parent - institution to visit Budapest (Hungary) in June, 2019. The author is recipient of a project from Indian Council of Agricultural Research to conduct research as Principal Investigator on "Bypassing dietary fats from Biohydrogenation for improving product quality in ruminants". He had guided and co-guided Post - graduate students as well as teaching for over three decades. He is a member of "Academic Council" of the above university, which is known as **Harbinger of Green revolution.**

Animal Nutrition and Feed Technology

Raman Rao Post-Doctoral Research Fellow (Canada)

Professor
Department of Animal Nutrition
College of Veterinary and Animal Sciences
G B Pant University of Agriculture & Technology
Sant Udham Singh Nagar, Pantnagar
Uttarakhand-263 145

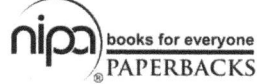

NIPA® GENX ELECTRONIC RESOURCES & SOLUTIONS P. LTD.
New Delhi-110 034

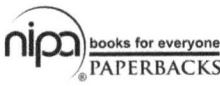

**NIPA® GENX ELECTRONIC
RESOURCES & SOLUTIONS P. LTD.**

101,103, Vikas Surya Plaza, CU Block
L.S.C. Market, Pitam Pura, New Delhi-110 034
Ph : +91 11 27341616, 27341717, 27341718
E-mail: newindiapublishingagency@gmail.com
www: www.nipabooks.com

For customer assistance, please contact
Phone: + 91-11-27 34 17 17
Fax: + 91-11- 27 34 16 16
E-Mail: feedbacks@nipabooks.com

© 2023, Publisher

ISBN: 978-81-19002-13-9

All rights reserved. No part of this publication may be reproduced, stored in a retrieval system or transmitted in any form or by any means, including electronic, mechanical, photocopying recording or otherwise without the prior written permission of the publisher or the copyright holder.

This book contains information obtained from authentic and highly reliable sources. Reasonable efforts have been made to publish reliable data and information, but the author/s, editor/s and publisher cannot assume responsibility for the validity, accuracy or completeness of all materials or information published herein or the consequences of their use. The work is published with the understanding that the publisher and author/s are not attempting to render any professional services. The author/s, editor/s and publisher have attempted to trace and acknowledge the copyright holders of all material reproduced in this publication and apologize to copyright holders if permission and/or acknowledgements to publish in this form have not been taken. If any copyrighted material has not been acknowledged, please write to us and let us know so that we may rectify the error, in subsequent reprints.

Trademark Notice: NIPA®, the NIPA® logos and their presentations (the way they are written/ presented) in this book are the trademarks of the publisher and hence may not be used without written permission, if copied or used without authorization, the infringer will be prosecuted as per law.

NIPA® also publishes books in a variety of electronic formats. Some content that appears in print may not be available in electronic books, and vice versa.

Composed and Designed by NIPA®.

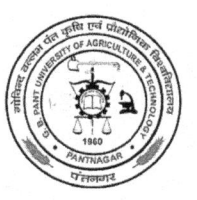

अनुसंधान निदेशालय
Directorate of Research
गो.ब. पन्त कृषि एवं प्रौद्योगिक विश्वविद्यालय, पन्तनगर
G.B. Pant University of Agriculture & Technology
Pantnagar-263 145
Distt. Udham Singh Nagar (Uttarakhand, INDIA)
Telephone (Off.): 05944-233363, Fax: 05944-233448 & 233473
Email: desgbpuat@gmail.com

Dr. S.N. Tiwari
Director Research

Foreword

Livestock plays an important role in the agrarian economy of most of the developing countries and more so in India because of small land holdings and a large percentage of rural population possessing no land. India has the world's best dairy buffaloes, draught cattle, carpet wool sheep and prolific goat breeds. The animal nutrition scientists have been carrying out systematic investigations on subsidiary feeds since Nineteen hundred fourty. The author has prepared this manuscript based on his past experiences and review of the knowledge on the subject available from the researches carried out at different places globally. He has very ably brought together valuable but widely dispersed information in this book. It is hoped that such knowledge will provide students, para-researchers and entrepreneurs engaged in compounded feed industry information on nutritive value of different feeds available today. The topics have full relevance in the present day animal nutrition scenario and definitely contribute in updating the knowledge of students, teachers and researchers. The compilation of varied aspects would be informative and possessed by each and everyone concerned in the field of animal nutrition. I wish the author success in the pursuit of his knowledge and I also wish the users a good luck and happy reading.

(S.N. Tiwari)

Preface

In its beginning, animal nutrition was an art. Infact, even today, many of the cattle feeders cling to the idea that "the eye of the master fattens his cattle". The foundations of animal nutrition were a blend of instinct, habit, experience, folklore and conjecture. Nutrition remained largely an art until the scientists entered the field and chemists described feeds in terms of chemical entities. The physiologists, endocrinologists and bacteriologists joined the team and this paved the way for demonstrating that the feeds are heterogeneous combination of nutrients. It was shown that most single feed is unbalanced in terms of an animal's requirements. The field of nutrition has moved forward at an accelerated pace, year by year, as the new knowledge accumulated. In preparing this manuscript, the general framework and character of the book established by seniors, have been preserved. The text presents the principles of nutrition and their applications to feeding practice. It not only presents facts but shows how many of these have been obtained, illustrating experimental methods which will continue to develop new facts in the future. Like other rapidly advancing fields, new discoveries in the science of nutrition, which add to our knowledge, inevitably cause some modification in ideas previously held. The literature citations have been made on the basis of their usefulness to those students who are the principal users of the text. Such a compilation has resulted in an unbalanced representation of nutrition research on a worldwide basis.

Suggestions received from teachers, including many former students is gratefully acknowledged. The author would welcome suggestions and healthy criticisms for future improvement.

Author

Contents

Foreword .... *v*
Preface .... *vii*

Section 01: Introduction

1. The Animal and its Feed 1
2. Categories of Animal Feeds 5
3. Importance of Nutrients 13
4. Digestion 29
5. Digestibility Determination of Feeds 33
6. Expressing the Energy Value of Feeds 35
7. Partition of Energy 37
8. Expressing the Protein Value of feeds 39
9. Feeding Standards 43
10. Fasting Heat Production 47
11. Animal Growth and Nutrition 53
12. Lactation 59
13. Examining Dairy Farm Management Closely 65
14. Feed Technology 89
15. Feeds for Sick and Old Animals 101
16. Pet Animal Nutrition 103
17. Principles of Zoo Mammal Nutrition 107
18. Feeding Zoo and Wild Animals 111

19. *Palo Podrido* Feed 117
20. Unconventional Feeds 125

Section 02: Applications

21. Basic Research 129
22. Formulation of Premix 133
23. Mechanic's of Feed Mixing of Feed Mixing 139
24. Automated Mill 143
25. Problems & Quarantine Measures in Feed Mill 149
26. Use of Computer on Feed Formulation 153
27. Codex Alimentarius 159
28. Biohydrogenation 165
29. Alkane Technology: An Extremely Powerful "User Friendly" Tool for Dairy Industry 169
30. Least Cost Accounting 171
31. Abnormal or Fertilized eggs of hen should not be marketed 173

    Appendices 181
    Appendix 1: Nutrient Reqirements of Livestock 181
    Appendix 2: Nutritive value of common feeds
        (Straws and green forages) 190

    Some Important Books 195

    Question and Answer 197

    Index 209

Section 01: Introduction

Introduction

Historical Aspects

Eighteenth century: Antoine Lavoisier, a French scientist was known to be as "Founder of science of nutrition". He established chemical basis of nutrition in his respiration experiments and introduced balance, thermometer in his studies. Alongwith Laplace, he designed a calorimeter through which it was demonstrated that respiration is the essential source of body heat. Even they started realizing that something is there like–carbohydrate, protein, fat and a need was felt for their investigation. But due to bad luck, French revolution took place and Lavoisier's career was ended by guillotine (be-heading). As a result, further studies on nutrition suffered a set back for several years.

Second half of 19th century: Babcock, an American dairy scientist observed that feeds of different sources were eaten by animals, but there was 'no way of knowing', what particular contribution each of those feeds was making to animal's needs. Therefore, he conceived the idea of trying the rations made up of entirely from a 'single plant'. He was criticized that his research was highly impractical. Later, his younger colleagues pursued this idea in another experiment. They planned their experiment more meticulously with more number of animals by feeding single crop rations. But, at that time, they could not conclude irrespective of their exhaustive chemical studies of feeds, excreta, tissues of dead calves. It was later on that the new discoveries provided the 'true answer'. Later based on this previous experience, "Purified diet method" was undertaken. Carbohydrate as pure starch, fat as pure lard or oil, protein as pure casein alongwith some minerals then known to be essential. It was revealed that there were certain other nutritional essentials which were very important.

Opening of 20th century: Research with artificial diets were repeated. Federich Hopkins began his career from Cambridge university in the field of bio-chemistry and nutrition. Early in his career, he isolated, purified and identified tryptophan and showed that 'Zein, a corn protein' could be improved nutritionally by adding this essential amino acid to it. He stated that no animal can survive on purified diet only, but there were certain other important factors which were highly vital for the animals. He coined the term "Accessory growth factors", which were essential for the prevention of deficiency diseases. For his above pioneering concepts of vitamins, he received **"Nobel prize for medicine in 1939"** alongwith Eijkman.

Animal Nutriton Research in Indian Sub-continent

As early as nineteen hundred twenties, a need for animal nutrition research was felt and hence, a laboratory of physiological chemist was established at Imperial Agriculture Research Institute (IARI), Pusa, Bihar in August, 1921 and was headed by Dr. F.J.Warth. In 1923, this laboratory was shifted to Imperial Institute of Animal Husbandry and Dairying at Bangalore. Later on, under the chairmanship of Lord Linithgow, Royal Commission on Agriculture, the animal nutrition division at Indian Veterinary Research Institute (IVRI) was established at Mukteshwar in 1935. This was the only principal centre of research in the field of animal nutrition. In early nineteen hundred fifties, National Dairy Research Institute, Karnal was established with a department on Dairy Cattle Nutrition and Physiology. In 1967, Indian Council of Agricultural Research (ICAR) had started research on utilization of agro – industrial by – products. In nineteen hundred seventies, the species wise (poultry, sheep, goat, buffalo, camel, equine) animal science institutes were established under the guidelines of ICAR. In nineteen hundred twenties and thirties, Dr. F.J. Warth initiated the evaluation of feeds and fodders at the Laboratory of Physiological Chemist, Bangalore. Further research on evaluation of feeds, Assam grasses and likewise were undertaken by Dr. K.C. Sen, Dr. S.K. Talapatra, Dr. N.D. Kehar. Lot of work on famine rations had been reported by Dr. N.D. Kehar.

Chapter 1

The Animal and its Feed

Nutrition involves various bio-chemical and physiological activities which transform feed elements into body elements. These feed elements are **nutrients** which are digested, absorbed, utilized to build and renew the components of the animal body. As a result, animal grows and produces-milk, eggs, wool with the help of energy so produced in the body. After weaning, most of our farm animals obtain all of their feed supply from plants. Barring carnivores, the plant kingdom is the original and essential source of all animal life, because plants are able to utilize the energy of the sun to build substances which nourish the animal. Plants make use of carbon dioxide, water and mineral salts to form carbohydrates, fats and proteins which are utilized in the life processes of animal body. Thus plants store and animals dissipate energy.

Plants and their parts

Animal body and plants contain the same substances but they differ in relative amounts. There are also much larger compositional differences among species than do animals. **Water** is the principal constituent of living plants as well as animal body. With the maturity of seed, water content decreases. The dry matter of plants consists principally of carbohydrates, which serve as both structural and reserve material, while in animals, protein comprises the structure of the soft tissues and fat is the reserve. Thus, *animal body contains only a trace of carbohydrate,* though occurring as much less than 1 per cent at any given moment, because it is constantly being formed and broken down in metablolism. Whereas, this is the principal constituent of most of the plant species. **Protein** is the main constituent of active tissues and thus leaves are much richer in this nutrient than are stems. Grass hays contain less protein than leguminous hays. When the plant matures, there is gradual movement of protein from the vegetative parts to the seed. Thus, the seed contains a higher percentage of protein than the rest of the plant, as in grains and stovers.

There is higher **fat** content in the leaves compared to the stems and generally is highest in the seeds, where this nutrient serves a condensed reserve of energy for later germination. The principal store of energy in most seeds is in the form of **carbohydrates**, but it is fat in oil-bearing seeds. Commercial sources of oil are extracted from these seeds, leaving oil meals as by products for animal feeding. Protein content is also higher in such oil-bearing seeds than is the cereal seeds. Carbohydrate is the principal constituent in all plant products, with the exception of oil-bearing seeds, even as it is in the plant as a whole. It occurs principally as starch, which is the reserve carbohydrate in seeds. While in stems and to a much lesser extent in leaves, a considerable proportion of it is present as cellulose, the principal structural carbohydrate. The outer coats of seeds also contain cellulose as a structural and protective element. The various parts of plants differ markedly in nutritive value according to their digestibility, because cellulose as crude fibre, is much less digestible than starch. Such feeds are classed as roughages, which are high in cellulose and thus of low digestibility. The seeds and the most of their by-products are classed as concentrates, to denote those low in crude fibre and hence highly digestible.

Mineral Matter

Mineral matter varies considerably in different plants as well as in the different plant parts. Similarly, distribution of mineral element differs markedly in plants than to those in animals. Calcium and phosphorus are the major inorganic components of animals, but they make-up a rather a small part of ash of plants, with the exception of legumes which are always rich in calcium. However, potassium and silicon are the main inorganic elements in plants. Calcium is primarily associated with the vegetative part of the plant, and the leaf is richer than stem. Seeds are low in calcium compared with the other parts of the plant, though oil-bearing seeds are higher than others. In contrast to calcium, phosphorus is richer in seeds than in the rest of the plant. Leaves are richer than stems. Soil and other cultural factors influence the calcium and phosphorus content of vegetative part of the plant.

By-Product Feeds

The familiar examples of the seed by-products are – the *bran, middling* arise from flour milling, gluten feed by-product of corn starch manufacture, and meals are the residues obtained from oil-bearing seeds. Their composition is usually very different from that of the seed or other material from which they arise. More of starch and less of digestible carbohydrates are present in the endosperm, but higher content of cellulose and related compounds comprise the seed coats as protective cover. They are also richer in protein, fat and mineral matter than the endosperm or the seed as a whole. The embryo is rich in protein and fat, but lowest of all in cellulose. Entire kernel, seed coats and embryo contain most of the vitamin content.

Industrial by-products

The by-product of wheat for animals is richer in protein, fat, mineral matter and vitamins than the entire kernel. But, kernel is somewhat less digestible because of the larger amount of the higher carbohydrates. It's the endosperm which provides the white flour for the human food. Oat mill by-product contains less than half as much protein and over twice as much fibre, because it consists mainly of the hull. It is therefore of low digestibility and nutritive value. On the other hand, mechanical or solvent extraction of soybeans, cotton seed to obtain their oils for human food or industrial use provides products that are highly digestible and of special value for their protein content. Similarly, many important feeds resulting from the processing of animal products are used in swine and poultry rations, for example, meat scraps, fish meal, milk by-products and many others. Such knowledge of the make-up, in terms of the different parts of the original material of by-product feeds, would be very helpful guide to their composition and feeding value.

Chapter 2

Categories of Animal Feeds

Livestock feeds have a variety of feed stuffs for feeding. Composition and characteristics differ even among closely related feeds. Also, cost and availability of such feeds at a particular place, makes the farmer to choose for practical feeding. Therefore, it becomes imperative to learn about such classes. Feeds may generally be classified according to the amount of a specific nutrient they provide in the ration. They may conveniently be divided into two general classes– roughages and concentrates. *Roughages* are bulky feeds containing more than 18 per cent crude fibre, but less than 60 per cent total digestible nutrients. Contrary to this, concentrates have less than 18 per cent fibre, but more than 60 per cent total digestible nutrients. Roughages may be further sub-divided into succulent and dry types. Whereas, *concentrates* are sub-divided into Energy or basal feeds having less than 20 per cent crude protein and Protein supplements having more than 20 per cent crude protein. Following feeds indicate the outlines of classification [Flow chart 1] of the conventional feeds into broad categories with examples.

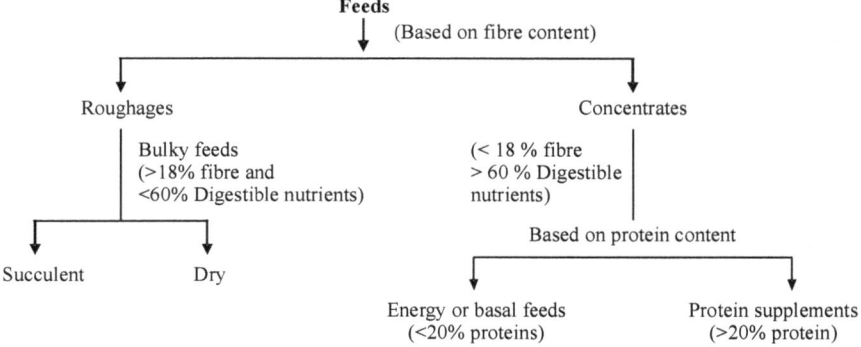

Flow chart 1 : Feeds for farm animals are classified according to amount of nutrient they provide in the diet.

Succulent Roughages

Pasture plants

Such feeds of herbivorous domestic animals are the natural plants which make up the most of the diet all through the time possible. There are two types of systems - continuous and rotational. In the continuous grazing, the animals are maintained on the same area. There is ideal stocking rate (i.e. animals per unit area) as well as grazing pressure. Therefore, there is balance between the growth of young herbage and its grazing (harvesting) by animals; hence they receive constant supply of nutritious herbage. Such pastures containing a wide variety of plants eg. Shrubs, grasses, herbaceous legumes, which are important for selective grazing. In the rotational grazing, both stocking rate and grazing pressure are high. The animals graze the pastures for short periods and most of the herbage of grsssland is harvested by animals and thereafter, lands are left to rest for longer periods of recovery.

Tree leaves

Generally, tree leaves are fed to sheep, goats, and during scarcity period to cattle too. Leaves of such trees contain fairly high content of crude protein and relatively low crude fibre, during early stages of their growth. There is a gradual decrease in protein content with an increase in crude fibre content with the maturity of plant. The tree leaves and shrubs are generally rich in calcium, but poor in phosphorus. *Indian kapok* or red silk cotton tree: This is grown for fine, lustrous material (*kapok*) obtained from the seed hairs. Flowers for human consumption. The leaves are about 8 cm long; are felted with star shaped hairs. Along with the twigs, these are lopped for fodder. *Fig*: A small spreading shrubby tree with large leaves. The leaves can be fed to cattle and should be collected as soon as the fruit has been harvested and before yellowing begins. *Coffee*: The dark, glossy green leaves of this bush are dried and included in the cattle concentrate. The leaves are palatable, without any unfavourable side effects. They were found to extend the lactation period. *Jack fruit:* Leaves are relished by ovines and cattle. The feeding is practiced in Kerala, Maharashtra, Orissa, West Bengal. *Banyan*: The leaves are relished by ovine and bovine both. *Peepal*: Commonly grown as an avenue tree. The leaves and branches are extensively lopped for fodder, though palatability and nutritive value of these leaves are not good. *Neem*: Normal livestock don't like but buffaloes found to consume about 5 kg / d. The tree is drought resistant and green throughout the year.

Cultivated forages

Legumes : These plant species have the unique ability to grow in symbiotic relationship with nitrogen fixing bacteria and for their drought resistance. The commonest legumes are as following:

Clover : Nutritionally, they are superior to grasses in protein and mineral content, particularly calcium, phosphorus, magnesium, copper, cobalt and their nutritive value falls less with age. The rates of reduction in particular size and of movement of particulate matter from the rumen are more rapid than with grass. It has been observed that cattle and sheep had consumed 20 per cent more dry matter than from grass of the same metabolizable energy content. Similar high voluntary intakes of dry matter have been obtained using other legumes. Berseem (Egyptian clover) is grown in India and Mediterranean area. It is valued for its rapid growth in winter season in the subtropics and for its good recovery after cutting or grazing. It has nutritive value very similar to that of Lucerne.

Lucerne (alpha alpha): It grows on its own. It is found in warm temperate areas and in many tropical and sub-tropical areas. The protein content is comparatively high and declines only slowly with maturity. They may be high in fibre, particularly in stem and at the late flowering stage, crude fibre may be high. Lucerne cultivars are distinguished by the time of flowering and for cold situations, early flowering types are recommended.

Silages : Controlled fermentation of a crop of high moisture content results in silage. This process is ensliling, carried out in silo for storage purpose. The process is essentially anaerobic, carried out by *Lactobacillus plantarum, Lactobacillus brevis, Clostridium butyricum*. Some grasses, some legumes or some non-legumes can be chopped and rapidly filled, pressed hard to prevent entry of air and then sealed for a period of 3 weeks.

Root crops and tubers : Turnips, fodder beet, sugarbeet or its pulp, carrot, potatoes, sweet potatoes are good for feeding farm animals.

Dry Roughages

Hay : Green crops (eg. Lucerne) are sun dried to reduce the moisture content to a level low enough to inhibit the action of plant and microbial enzymes. eg. Some legumes, some non-legumes, some cereals crops etc.

Straws and related by-products : Stems and leaves of most cereal crops and some legumes after the removal of the ripe seeds by threshing are called straws. During threshing, husk or glumes of the seed are separated from the grain. Straws of wheat, paddy, barley, oat, maize, rye, beans, peas, Corn cobs, Cotton seed hulls are fed to ruminants with highly succulent roughage to avoid nutritional disorder bloat.

Energy (Basal) Feeds

Cereal grains : Members of Gramineae family are cultivated for their seeds. They have been termed as 'cereal' (eg. maize, corn, barley, oats, sorghum). These grains are essentially carbohydrate concentrates. Grannular starch is the main component which is accumulated in the endosperm. The dry matter content of the grain is about 800 g/kg on an average. Embryo and aleurone layer have proteins. It has been shown that cereal proteins are in the order of oat > maize > or wheat for promoting chick growth. Embryo or germ contains more oil than the endosperm and these are unsaturated linoleic and oleic fatty acids, hence produce a soft body fat in the swine and poultry. Harvested grain contains highest crude fibre content in husk or hull formed from the fused glumes of oat or rice and lowest in the denuded grains – wheat and maize. Cereals are deficient in calcium, but phosphorus is high as phytic acid, concentrated in the aleurone layer. Cereal phytates have the property of being able to bind dietary calcium, magnesium and hence prevent their absorption from the gut. With the exception of yellow maize, grains are deficient in vitamin D, pro-vitamin A. They are good sources of vitamin E and Thiamin but low content of riboflavin. Most of the vitamins are concentrated in aleurone layer and the germ of the grain. Calves, swine and poultry depend upon cereal grains for their main source of energy.

Mill by-products of cereal grains

Wheat by-products: Cryopsis of wheat comprises of 3 per cent germ, 15 per cent bran or seed coat and 82 per cent endosperm. After milling, bran coat is released from the endosperm. Coarse wheat feed, or bran contains more fibre and less protein than fine wheat feed and has always been a popular feed for horses. The germ or embryo is very rich in protein, low in fibre and excellent source of thiamin and vitamin E. It may be collected separately or may be allowed to flow on the fine wheat feed by-product. All classes of farm animals may be safely fed with fine wheat feed.

Oat by-products

Oat husks or hulls: Seventy per cent of oat husks or hulls form the total main by-product. Oat hulls are of very low feeding value, being little better than oat straw. Their crude protein or crude fibre content is very low for ruminants.

- *Oat dust*: This is rich in kernel material including kernel hairs removed from the grain during brushing. It has a pretty good amount of protein content.
- *Meal seeds:* These consist of slivers (a long thin piece split off) of husk and fragments of kernels approximately in equal proportion.
- *Oat feed:* It has combination of oat hulls, oat dust in 4 to 1 proportion. This feed is fairly better than the hulls in feeding value.

Barley by-products

Malt culms: Consist of plumule and radical of barley and are rich in crude protein. Because of their fibrous nature, feeding is restricted to ruminants and horses. Due to presence of asparagine amino acid, it has bitter flavor, which forms one third of protein. That is why it is mixed with other feed so that it may be readily acceptable. A related by – product is "malt residual pellets", which comprise malt culms and other malt screenings. These have low fibre but high starch contents than plain malt culms, giving a slightly high energy for ruminants.

Brewers' grains (draff): This by – product contains barley residue, maize and rice residues and hence, composition is highly variable. This product is fed to sheep, cattle, horses as such or preserved as silage.

Spent hops: A fibrous product comparable to poor hay in nutritive value. Due to bitter flavor, is less palatable.

Dried brewers' yeast: It's a protein rich concentrate. Its highly digestible and fed to all classes of farm animals. Protein is of fairly high nutritive value and favoured for feeding swine and poultry. It's a valuable source of many of the 'B' group of vitamins and relatively rich in phosphorus but has low calcium.

Protein concentrates : After extraction of the greater part of the oil from oil seeds, residues of oil seed cakes and meals are left, which are rich in protein. Most of such residues are highly valuable for farm animals. These oil seed meals are also high in protein, phosphorous content but low in calcium content. They may furnish useful amounts of B – vitamins but are poor sources of carotene and vitamin E.

Beans: Broad bean, horse bean or Windsor bean is the main variety including kidney, field, garden or haricot beans. They are good sources of protein with high lysine content and good sources of energy, but have low contents of calcium. There is little or no carotene or vitamin C in beans but may contain significant amounts thiamin, niacin and riboflavin. They are primarily of good quality protein. This is refection of the amino acid composition characterized by high lysine content similar to that of fish meal protein. Common animal and vegetable proteins do have more cystine and methionine than these beans. These are fed to all major classes of farm animals, usually cracked, kibbed or coarsely ground form. But, whole beans are quite satisfactory for older ruminants. Ground beans would be good for sow, weaner and fattening diets but not in creep feeds. Beans may be replaced with soybean meal for poultry alongwith adequate methionine.

Peas: Similar to beans, Peas (for example Chick pea) are basically similar but have lower contents of crude protein and crude fibre. Compared to beans, they have slightly higher oil content but the degree of saturation is similar. Primarily, peas are considered as a source of protein with better balance of amino acids, having higher contents of lysine, methionine and cystine, though methionine is still the main limiting amino acids. They are able to replace soybean meal for poultry and swine diets, whereas beans are largely confined to ruminant dites. For compounding feeds, they make an important ingredient alongwith beans.

Animal protein concentrates: When the simple-stomached animals are fed on all-vegetable-protein diet, they suffer deficiency of certain indispensable amino acids. Therefore, animal protein sources are included in conjunction with another animal or vegetable protein to complement and adequately make good the deficiency of such amino acids. In addition, they often make a significant contribution to the animal's mineral nutrition as well as supplying various vitamins of B-complex. Moreover, these animal products are given in limited quantities to farm animals, because they are expensive and hence their large scale use is uneconomic.

Meat meal: This feed contains more protein relative to meat and bone meal, whereas, reverse is the situation with ash content in these two. Meat and bone meal is an excellent source of Ca, P and Mn. Fat content is variable and both are good sources of B-complex, particularly choline, riboflavin, cyanocobalmine and nicotinamide. Meat by-products may be used for supplementing lysine content.

Fish meal: These are having proteins in appreciable amounts and are rich in lysine, cystine, methionine and tryptophan. Therefore, this is a valuable supplement to cereal-based diets where they have more proportion of maize. This meal contains high content of Ca, P, Mn, Fe, I and very good source of B – complex vitamins-riboflavin, choline, cyanocobalamine as well as Animal Proein Factor (APF). Energy is largely a refection of the oil content.

Blood meal: This meal is one of the richest source of lysine and a rich source of arginine, methionin, cystine and leucine. Due to poor balance of amino acids, its biological value is low and also it has a low digestibility. This feed may be fed to older poultry.

Hydrolysed feather meal: This meal has a high protein content, which may be included in the diet gradually to combat low palatability. *Salmonella* contamination should be checked periodically.

Single cell protein: Yeast and bacteria grow very quickly, can double their cell mass in three to four hours. Such process was adopted for large scale industrial production of proteins from cereal grains, sugarcane, sugar beet, their by-products, hydrolysates from wood and plants. *Pseudomonas* sp., *Saccharomyces* sp., *Candida* sp. are helpful for such fermentation.

Non-protein compounds as protein sources: These compounds are very good sources of nitrogen for microbial protein synthesis in ruminants. Urea had been very familiar among other such compounds, which is widely used with regard to cost, convenience and palatability.

Milk products

Whole milk: Cow milk contains on an average 85 % water, 15 % dry matter of total solids-of which about 38 % is fat and remainder solids not fat (SNF). The latter one contains 33 % protein including casein, 47 % lactose and 8 % ash. There is deficiency of sulphur containing amino acids-cysteine, cystine, methionine but fortunately b-lactoglobulin is rich in these acids so that biological value is 0.85. The most economical use of the whole milk is in supplemental poor quality of proteins analogous to cereals. Such replacement is better than using meat or fish products. Milk is also good source of vitamin A, thiamin, riboflavin and some vitamin B_{12}. Whole milk is fed to such calves, lambs, young dairy and bull calves as well as those prepared for competition. Two main products are valuable – Skim milk and whey.

Skim milk: Cream residue is separated from milk by centrifugal force and hence, total fat content is low. Removal of fat results in low fat soluble vitamins but there is concentration of solid not fat (SNF). Skim milk is mainly used as protein supplement for simple stomached animals, particularly effective in making good amino acid deficiencies of young swine.

Whey: During cheese making, milk is treated with rennet and casein is precipitated, which carries down with it most of the fat and about half of the calcium and phosphorus. The left - over is called whey. Most of the protein is β-lactoglobulin and is very good quality which may be fed to swine. Unlike skim milk, whey proteins do not clot in the stomachs, however high rates of inclusion may cause digestive problem.

Miscellaneous

There are certain non – nutritive products which are stimulant in the feeding to non – ruminants. If not included in their diet, there is no loss but they have been observed to be certainly beneficial for health of the animal. Antibiotics: tetracycline, aureomycin, penicillin etc.; Antioxidants: Butylated hydroxyl toluene (BHT); Buffers; Colours and flavours; Enzymes; Hormones; Medicines: Coccidiostat is invariably added whether the problem is there or not.; Emulsifying agents: fats etc.

Chapter 3

Importance of Nutrients

There are six nutrients which are very important to animal body and they are – Carbohydrates, Lipids, Proteins, Minerals, Vitamins and water.

Carbohydrates: These are polyhydroxy aldehyde or ketone as in monosaccharide or polymers in oligo or polysaccharides. The question arises whether carbohydrate is a dietary essential !!! **Carbohydrate** may not be dietary essential but it is definitely metabolically essential. The organic compounds – fats, proteins are oxidized only in the presence of carbohydrates. Carbohydrates are the structural components of DNA, RNA, and some other vital organic molecules. Although less than 1% is present in the human body (because constantly being formed and broken down in metabolism), yet without the presence of this carbohydrate, the existence of living creature is at stake.

Carbohydrate in the form of glucose primarily provides energy in the body and excess amount of carbohydrate is stored as glycogen in the liver and muscle. More than fifty per cent of the energy value of the diet is provided by carbohydrate.

Glucose + $6O_2$ → $6 CO_2$ + $6H_2O$ + ΔE (675 k.cal)

They also exhibit protein sparing action because proteins are mainly required for tissue-building i.e. general wear and tear in the body. If there is any emergency, say animal is deficient in calories of the diet, then it will use adipose and protein tissues. It is said that proteins and fats are burnt or oxidized in the flame of carbohydrate. It means that certain intermediary compounds of glucose oxidation through krebs cycle are absolutely necessary for oxidation of proteins and fats. Again, in any emergency, if glucose level of the body goes down, fats and proteins take over and they get metabolized faster than the animal body can take care of the intermediate products. However, ketone bodies-acetone, acetoacetate, β-hydroxy butyrate appear in the urine. In addition to above, monosaccharides are very important (vital) structural components of many compounds which regulate metabolism. Among these are DNA, RNA for transfer of genetic information of the cell, which contain ribose and deoxy ribose sugars. Glucuronic acid occurs in the liver and this combines with toxic chemicals and bacterial by-products and hence acts as detoxifying agent.

Hyluronic acid (a disaccharide) forms matrix of connective tissue. Heparin, a muco polysaccharide, is very important anticoagulant. Chondroitin sulfates are present in cartilage, bone, skin and tendon. Glycosides are widely distributed thoughout the plant kingdom and a number of them have been used as drugs for animals.

Lipids: These are important constituents of plant and animal tissue and these can be extractable from biological materials with the usual fat solvents eg. Ether, chloroform, benzene, carbon tetrachloride, acetone etc. The lipid metabolism is in dynamic state. There is constant mobilization and transportation of fatty acids from the depots. Some portion of absorbed fatty acids are degraded in the same way, while others are combined with glycerol transported back to depots. All these reactions are so balanced that mixtures of fatty acids in the depots, blood and organs tend to remain at equilibrium condition.

Lipids are the most concentrated form of stored energy in animal kingdom, because they provide 2.25 times per unit more energy than carbohydrate. They provide insulation for vital organs protecting them from mechanical shock and also maintain body temperature. The cell membranes have phospholipids eg. Erythrocytes. Prostaglandins exhibit hormonal activities. Essential fatty acids – linoleic, linolenic and arachidonic acids show deficiency symptoms in their absence. Lipid also delays hunger because it requires loger time to pass through stomach than carbohydrate or protein. They also help in lubrication.

Proteins: In 1938, a Dutch chemist – G.J.Mulder described certain organic material which is unquestionably the most important of all known substances in the organic kingdom, without which, no life appears possible on our planet. He also used the term protein (In Greek, proteios mens the first) to describe these vital compounds. Proteins are major structural components of animal tissue, just as cellulose provides for the plants. Proteins are components of skin, hair, wool, eggs, feathers, nails, horns, hoofs, muscles, tendons, connective tissue and supporting tissue such as cartilage. In addition, proteins are involved in communication (nerves), defense (antibodies), metabolic regulation (hormones), biochemical catalysts (enzymes) and oxygen transport (haemoglobin). For wear - tear or general maintenance of the body, proteins are constantly in demand. Lipid and carbohydrates are stored by the body as energy reserves, but proteins are not stored to any appreciable extent. It is possible for animals to survive for a short period of time on a diet consisting of proteins, vitamins and minerals, but an animal may not survive over the same period of time on protein-free diet containing lipids, carbohydrates, vitamins and minerals.

Proteins or amino acids are important for the synthesis of cell protoplasm. During metabolism, old tissues are worn out and new tissues are synthesized.

They also help in the synthesis of bile acids. All the enzymes are proteins, so we can imagine the importance. Milk proteins, antibodies eg. Colustrum (γ globulins), melanin (skin pigment), rhodopsin (visual pigment in eye) are of high significance.

Minerals

The mineral is an essential element which has a metabolic role in the body and if not provided in the diet, can cause deficiency symptoms, which can be prevented by adding that element to the diet. Animal body contains about 3 % minerals, which are constant constituents of animal tissues. Classification is based on the amount required by the animals. Major elements are required in large amounts and are expressed in percentage, whereas minor or trace elements are required in small amounts and hence expressed in parts per million or billion or even trillion. They exhibit some very important functions-catalytic (some are bound to enzymes), chelating (in chlorophyll, haemoglobin, vitamin B_{12}, cytochromes), electrochemical (for maintaining osmotic pressure and acid – base balance in the blood), structural (in the skeleton), as a constituent (in thyroxine, vitamin B_{12}, haemoglobin) and multiple roles too. Metabolic role, deficiency or toxic problem and sources have been given in the Table 1.

Vitamins

When animals are maintained on a chemically defined diet containing only purified proteins, carbohydrates, fats and necessary minerals, it is not possible to sustain life. Certain additional factors present in natural feeds, which are required only in minute amounts but are necessary. These are 'accessory growth factors' which cannot be synthesized by the host and therefore, must be obtained either from the diet or from the microbes of the intestinal tract. Ascorbic acid, for example, is a vitamin for man and other primates-monkey, guinea pig, and bat. This may be called a hormone in all animals, because they are capable of biosynthesizing. Chemical nature, metabolic role, deficiency problems and sources have been given in the Tables 2 & 3.

Water

Animal body is composed of two thirds water (intra and extra cellular fluids) and that a feed is any substance used by the body for building tissue, it is obvious that water is very important nutrient. Experiments have shown that animals may live for 100 days without organic feed, but they may die within 5 to 10 days, when deprived off water. Cell rigidity and elasticity imparts a definite form to body, which may be changed by the liquid content of the cell. Due to its high dielectric constant, oppositely charged ions can co-exist in water without much interference. Hydrolysis is an important chemical process in digestion and other metabolism, where H^+ and OH^- ions of water are introduced into bigger molecules and then these bigger molecules are broken down into smaller units. Lubrication is yet another important function where water prevents friction or drying in joint, conjunctiva, mouth, pleura surrounding lungs, other soft organs. Body heat regulation is carried out due to certain properties-for example, due to high specific heat of water can absorb large quantity of heat than any other liquid. Similarly, due to high heat conducting power, water can carry away heat from the site of production and distributing it throughout body. Because of these two properties, water acts as a buffer. Yet another due to such property, highest latent heat of evaporation, the body is able to get-rid off heat through urine and faeces and by evaporation from skin, lungs or tongue. Oxygen and carbon dioxide are soluble in water, hence gaseous exchange takes place in the tissues, for example, fish. The "aqueous humour" of eye helps to keep up the "shape" and "elasticity" of the eye-ball and acts as a refractive medium.

Importance of Nutrients

Table 1: Metabolic role in body, deficiency symptoms and sources of mineral elements

Major minerals:

Mineral	Metabolic role in the body	Deficiency symptoms.	Sources
Ca	• Important constituent of skeleton, cells, fluids. • Presence is important for enzyme systems. • Role in the transmission of nerve impulses. • Important for muscle contraction. • Coagulation of blood. • Role in the egg shell formation of poultry.	• In farm animals: In young: Rickets In adult : Osteomalacia. [Imbalance of Ca & P in bone formation in above both] * In dairy cows (lactating): Milk fever [paralysis, unconsciousness]. * In poultry: Egg production goes down, thin egg shells.	• Legumes, fish meal, bone meal, dicalcium phosphates. • Oyster shells, • Dicalcium phosphate.
P	• Occurs in bones, phosphoproteins, nucleic acid, phospholipids. • Role in carbohydrate metabolism.	• In farm animals: In young: Rickets In adult : Osteomalacia. [Imbalance of Ca & P in bone formation in above both] • In cattle: PICA, where appetite goes down. • In dairy cows: milk yield goes down.	In the decreasing order (plant origin): Wheat bran > cotton seed meal > linseed meal. Animal origin: Meat scraps, milk.
K	• Regulation of acid - base & osmotic balance. • Important intra - cellular cation. • Important for nerve & muscle excitation. • Role in carbohydrate metabolism.	• No deficiency as such, because potassium content of plants is very high. • But, excess may interfere with Mg metabolism.	Pastures.

Element	Functions	Deficiency/Symptoms	Sources
Na	- Like K, Regulation of acid – base & osmotic balance. - Important extra – cellular cation of blood plasma and other extra cellular fluids.	- In farm animals: slow growth.	- Marine origin feeds.
Cl	- Associated with Na & K Regulation of acid – base & osmotic balance. - Role in gastric juice secretion (HCl) in stomach. - Excreted in urine, perspiration (sweat).	- So long as salt is there in diet, no deficiency at all. Even if deficiency occurs, that will not be immediate. - In farm animals: Appetite goes down, weight loss. - In poultry: Cannibalism (feather picking). - Toxic level: Thirst increases, muscular weakness, Edema (fluids in extra – cellular spaces).	- Fish meal. - Meat meal. - NaCl (common salt) - Limestone, oyster shells.
S	- Two forms – (a) Inorganic: as SO_4 ions in blood; (b) Organic: mostly as **Protein** (cysteine, cystine, methionine); **Vitamin:** thiamine, biotin; **Hormone:** insulin; Wool (sheep): Rich in cystine (4 %).	- **No deficiency at all**, because deficiency of sulfur would mean, a deficiency of protein and this is not possible.	- Proteins - Na_2SO_4.
Mg	- Associated with Ca & P. - 70 % of Mg: present in the skeleton. - Rest: soft tissues and fluids. - Enzyme activator: Decarboxylases & phosphatases.	- In ruminants: Hypo – magnesaemic Tetany: nervousness & staggering gait. - The problem starts when animal grazes on the young succulent pastures very low in Mg & hence Tetany develops. - It develops so rapidly that Mg reserves of the body can not be mobilized rapidly. - As a result, blood Mg levl goes down, bone depletion continues gradually. In acute stage, animal may die.	- Wheat bran - Protein concentrates.

Trace minerals:

Element	Functions	Deficiency/Symptoms	Sources
Fe	- > 90 % combines with haemoglobin. - Rest: (a) Transferin: For transport of iron in blood serum; (b). Ferritin: As storage in spleen, liver, bone - marrow; (c) Enzyme component: cytochromes, flavoproteins.	- In farm animals: Anaemia. - In poultry: egg production drops. - Excess Fe: P utilization drops.	- Legumes - Green leafy plant materials.

Importance of Nutrients

Element	Functions	Deficiency / Toxicity	Sources
Cu	• Helps in haemoglobin formation & R.B.C. production. • As a component of cytochrome oxidase. • Turacin: a pigment found in feather, wool, hair.	• In general: Anaemia • Excess Cu: Teart problem, Cu poisoning, may lead to death of the animal.	• Seeds & seed by-product.
Co	• Structural component of vitamin B_{12}. • Very important in propionic acid metabolism. Coenzyme B_{12} – dependent methylmalonyl - Co A mutase is responsible for the conversion of methyl malonyl Co A to succinyl Co A.	• In ruminants, Pining problem, where vitamin B_{12} drops, because pasture would be low in Co. After several months, appetite goes down, weight loss and then anaemia.	• Spray of $CoSO_4$ on the plants.
I	• Structural component of Thyroxine hormone. • Stimulates egg production in poultry.	• Goitre: swelling of neck. • Toxic level: Embryonic death in poultry. • No deficiency in farm animals.	• Fish meal, • Marine weeds.
Mn	• Occurs mainly in liver. • Enzyme activator, mainly bone phosphatase (resembles Mg).	• In poultry: Perosis or slipped tendon, where leg bones are affected in chicks.	• Rice bran. • Wheat offals.
Zn	• Storage is in bones (unlike other trace minerals, which are in liver). • Respiratory Enzyme activator – carbonic anhydrase in R.B.C., where removes CO_2.	• In non – ruminants (swin & poultry): Parakeratosis (reddening of skin & also, bone abnormality, hence storage is affected.	• Yeast • Sprouting grains.
Mo	• Has a role in purine metabolism (xanthine oxidase enzyme). • Helps in other enzymes – nitrate reductase, bacterial dehydrogenase.	• No deficiency but **Toxic role**: Teart prolem as in Cu, where Cu – retention drops.	• No need, because already toxic. Natural feeds are sufficient.
Se	• No role of its own, but in combination of vitamin E, prevents Muscular dystrophy (cattle) & Encephalomalcia (chicks).	• No deficiency but **Toxic role**: Its like Mo – Alkali disease or Blind staggers; where loss of hair in the tails, hoof are abnormal too.	• No need.
F	• In late 1930's, it was discovered that the fluoride ion can play a significant role in the prevention of human dental caries.	• No deficiency, but toxic level is poisonous, because causes Flurosis.	• Animals should not be in the vicinity of industrial polluted wastes and water.

- Most plant species have a limited capacity to absorb fluorine from the soil, even when fluoride – containing fertilizers are applied. Certain plant species, notably the **tea plant** and the **Camellia** are exceptional in this respect.
- Dental defects and some loss of appetite may appear with the significant rise in plasma fluoride levels. Anaemia has also been reported. Incisors become pitted and molars abraded. There may also be exposure of pulp cavities due to fracture or wear even **mottled enamel**.
- Teeth are pitted, pulp cavities are exposed, teeth become sensitive to cold water, appetite goes down, slow growth, bone deformity.
- The ingestion of toxic or potentially toxic amounts of fluorine by farm animals occurs most commonly in restricted areas adjacent to industrial plants or fluoride dusts which contaminate the soil, the herbage and water consumed by the animals.

Cd

- There is similarity between the atomic structure and chemical behavior of Cd and Zn ; high concentration of Cd that occurs in kidney.
- A protein compound was isolated, which contained as much as 5.9 % Cd and 2.2 % Zn from equine renal cortex and named "Metallothionein". Later, this compound was also found in human kidney and liver.
- Cd is virtually absent in new born's kidney but accumulates for next five decades.
- Cd is a Zn antimetabolite. Such antagonism as well as important interactions between Cd and Cu and Fe are apparent from several animal studies.
- A relationship between Cd and human **hypertension** had been postulated.
- Epidemiological evidence showed that Cd is a causal factor in hypertension.
- It is highly concentrated in wheat – germ, milled rice.
- The Cd content of the ash of the polished rice was 4 times that of the unpolished.
- Oysters are exceptionally rich in Cd, as are in Zn (3 – 4 ppm Cd wet weight).

Importance of Nutrients

Cr
- In 1911, it was shown to be up–taken by plants from soils.
- It was reported to be constituent of proteolytic enzymes and to be essential for their function.
- It is cofactor with insulin necessary for normal glucose utilization, for growth and longevity in rats and mice.
- **Trivalent** chromium is poorly absorbed and appears mainly in the faeces. Chromic oxide is so insoluble that it had found wide application as a **'marker'** for determining the digestibility of components of the diet and feed intakes by grazing stock.
- Anionic **hexavalent** chromium is better absorbed and hence, readily passes through the membrane of red blood corpuscles and becomes bound to the globins' fraction of hemoglobin.
- ^{51}Cr is labelled to erythrocytes, platelets and plasma proteins to determine their life–span or survival time.
- Tissue – uptake is quite rapid and absorbed / injected Cr is excreted mainly in urine with small amounts being lost in the bile and small intestine and possibly through the skin.

- Impaired growth, longevity and disturbances in glucose, lipid and protein metabolism.
- Rats on diets low in protein and chromium (< 0.1 ppm) also develop corneal lesion in the eyes.

- Chromium resembles most trace elements in being concentrated in the branny layers and germ of cereal grains.
- Chromium is lost in the process of sugar refining, so that white sugars contain very little, compared to the amounts in brown or raw sugar.
- In some areas, the drinking water (or potable) can be a significant source of chromium.

V
- V occurs in human enamel, dentin and may exchange with P.
- V exists in the blood as vanadium protein compound – Hemovanadium in Ascidian worm. This protein can't act as an oxygen carrier.

- It exhibited diarrhea as well as mortality in animals.
- Not toxic to human but may cause some cramps and diarrhea at the larger dose level. The amounts were observed in the urine.

- Blue – green alga: **Anabaena**. V can partially replace Mo for N – fixation by Azatobactor.

	- V salts are poorly absorbed from alimentary canal and appear mostly in the faeces.
- V inhibits synthesis of cholesterol from acetate as well as from mevalonic acid but not from squalene.	- Vanadium reduces Coenzyme A and Coenzyme Q levels in rats, that is, mammalian enzyme system.	
Ni	- Ni content of human female hair is significantly higher than males.
- Cow's milk and colostrum have average level of about **0.08 ppb Ni**.
- Ni activates several enzyme systems, eg. Arginase, Trypsin, Carboxylase, acetyl coenzyme A synthetase.
- It plays a role in pigmentation in several species of animals: fish, birds and insects. There is strong affinity of melanin and its precursors for metals, that colour depends upon specific metals, which are transmitted as genes.
- It is consistently present in RNA from diverse sources in concentrations many times higher than in the native material from which the RNA is isolated.	- Implicated as a **pulmonary carcinogen** in tobacco smoke.
- Serum nickel increases in Myocardial infarction.
- Growth and appetite reduced in young growing mice.
- Enzyme activity goes down, eg. Cytochrome oxidase (liver); Malic dehydrogenase (kidney).	- Vegetarian diets will supply much more nickel than non – vegetarian diets, because of higher content of foods of plant origin.
- Whole grains, vegetables, fruits, tubers.
- Oysters.
Sn	- It is widely but irregularly distributed in the biosphere.
- A significant growth effect in rats maintained on purified amino acid diets. This suggests that tin is an essential trace element for mammals.
- Tin was demonstrated in some but not all human and animal tissues examined – human teeth, spinal fluid as well as human and cow's milk.	- Ingested tin has a low toxicity, no doubt due in part to its poor absorption and retention in the tissues.
- The higher consumption of canned foods and juices could account at least in part, for their higher body burden of tin.	- Little interest shown in the tin content of forage and intakes of Sn by farm animals. This may merely mean that the concentrations are below the limits of detection of the methods employed.

Importance of Nutrients

- Little or no tin was found in the tissues of still born infants. This suggests that this element does not readily cross the placental barrier, but **"arrives in tissues shortly after birth, de novo"**.
- Large amounts of tin – can accumulate in foods in contact with tin plate, particularly when non – lacquered. Storage of canned tin, presumably due to corrosion starting from defects in the lacquer.

As

- The word arsenic has become so identified with **"poison"** in the public mind that the more valuable aspects of arsenic have tended to be obscured.
- Arsenic is widely distributed in the biosphere. It occurs in the air of areas where coal is burnt, particularly near smelters and refineries, in sea water, public water supplies [to the extent of **3 ppb**; detected by **"Neutron activation analysis"**]. Higher levels in soils can result from continued use of arsenical sprays.
- Arsenic is observed fairly well in the skin, nails, toes, hair.
- The beneficial effects of various organic arsenicals on the growth, health and feed efficiency of poultry and swine have been thoroughly established.
- Arsenic acids were recognized as Coccidiostats and growth stimulants for swine and poultry.
- Precise mechanism of action is unknown. However, arsenic closely resembles that of antibiotics and is to some extent complementary to it.
- It has a possible role as an anti-thyroid agent.
- Human hair: The arsenic content of hair has excited considerable interest because of its value in the diagnosis of **arsenic poisoning**. Normal hair always contains arsenic in small amounts, but increases by excessive intakes. Male and female hair differ significantly in arsenic content.
- It is said that two hair samples of Napolean First revealed high levels of arsenic. Hence, it is presumed that he might have suffered from arsenic poisoning during his last days on St. Helena. But it could not be confirmed at that time.
- Lower limit of spectrographic method was 10 ppm.
- **Lichens** were found to concentrate this element, so that those growing on silicic rocks contained the remarkably high mean level and those on ultrabasic rocks.
- Most human foods rarely exceed 1 ppm As (as fresh) and this applies to fruits, vegetables, cereal products, meats and dairy products.
- By contrast, foods of marine origin are very much richer in arsenic.
- Bony fish, oyster, mussels, prawns, shrimps have pretty well detectable amounts.

Table 2: Chemical nature, sources, metabolic role and deficiency symptoms of fat soluble vitamins.

Attributes	Vitamin A	Vitamin D	Vitamin E	Vitamin K	Vitamin C
Chemical nature	• Pale yellow crystalline solid, soluble in fat solvents. • Readily destroyed by light or air.	• There are 10 different forms, but only 2 are naturally occurring – D_2 (Ergo-Calciferol) and D_3 (chole – calciferol).	• There are 8 naturally occurring forms ÷ into 2 groups – (a) Saturated: $\alpha,\beta,\gamma,\delta$ Tocopherols. α is the most biologically active form (b) Unsaturated: $\alpha,\beta,\gamma,\delta$ Tocotrienols. This α form is 25 % that of α saturated form.	• Also known as Koagulation or K – factor (in foreign language at the place of discovery). • Ruminants can synthesize. • Two forms: K_1 (Naturally occurring) and K_2 (bacterial) • Rapidly destroyed on exposure to sun – light.	• Chemically known as l. – Ascorbic acid. • This is synthesized by ruminants and poultry birds, hence not required. • Rapidly destroyed on exposure to light or air.
Sources	• Liver (because of storage). • All carotene containing plant sources, eg. Carrot, green leafy plant materials.	• D_2 : Sun – dried roughages and dead leaves of growing plants. • D_3 : Some fish, cod – liver oil, egg –yolk, colustrum.	• Green fodders • Young grasses (not matured ones). • Cereal grains. • Animal sources are poor in vitamin E	• K_1: Green leafy material, Lucerne, cabbage. Animal sources: Egg yolk, fish meal. • K_2 (bacteria)	• Citrus fruits, green succulent leafy vegetables. • Commercially are also available.

Importance of Nutrients

	Vitamin A	Vitamin D	Vitamin E	Vitamin K	Vitamin C
Metabolic role.	• Vitamin A (*trans*) retinol is inactive gets oxidized in, dim light to retinal (*trans*) & then to its isomer *cis* form. Now this cis form + opsin → rhodopsin photo receptor. • When light falls on retina, *cis* → *trans* & released from opsin. This conversion results in transmission of an impulse along the optic nerve to brain. • Protects epithelial cells of mucous membranes.	• Helps in calcium absorption. • Has a role in growth, deposition of Ca and P on bones. • Helps in para-thyroid activity.	• Biological anti-oxidant. • Prevents the oxidation of unsaturated fatty acids. • Acts as hydrogen donor in the hydrogen transferring systems.	• Helps in blood clotting for the formation of prothrombin. • Has a role in electron transport chain.	• Has a role in oxidation-reduction mechanisms. • Has a role only in man and other primates: monkey, guinea pig, bat.
Deficiency symptoms: a) Farm animals.	• Rough hair, scaly skin. • Night blindness • Xerophthalmia (drying of conjuciva).	• In young animals: Rickets. • In older animals: Osteomalacia	• Muscular dystrophy, where circulatory & respiratory problems associated.	• No deficiency in farm animals. Because, synthesized by rumen microbes. • Moreover, all green leafy materials are rich in vitamin K.	• No deficiency in farm animals. • Scurvy only in primates and humans.

b)	Swine	• Night blindness • Xerophthalmia.	• Paralysis.	• Nil.	• Nil.
c)	Poultry	• High mortality rate. • Staggering gait.	• Egg production goes down. • Imbalance of Ca & P metabolism.	• Fatal sycope (heart muscle is affected, may lead to death of the animal). • Encephalomalacia.	• Delayed clotting. Grasses be included in the ration.

Note: For the sake of convenience of viewing at a glance, the water soluble vitamin C has also been included here.

Table 3: Chemical nature, metabolic role, deficiency symptoms and sources of vitamin B – complex.

Vitamin	Chemical nature	Metabolic role	Deficiency symptoms	Sources
Thiamine	Thiamine di phosphate (TPP) form is found in animal tissue.	• Oxidative decarboxylation of pyruvic acid. • Participation in Hexose Mono Phosphate (HMP) shunt pathway	• In farm animals: Nervous disorders, Bere – beri. • In poultry: Polyneuritis.	• Liver, • Yeast, • Germinating grains.
Riboflavin	Structural component of flavoproteins.	• Biosynthesis of flavin nucleotides (FMN, FAD coenzymes) • Role in oxidation – reduction reactions.	• In farm animals: Growth goes down, eye – diseases. • In chicks: Curled – toe – paralysis.	• Liver, • Yeast, • Green leafy crops.
Nicotinamide	Its formed from Tryptophan.	• Component of pyridmine nucleotide (NAD / NADP).	• In farm animals: Growth goes down. • Dermatitis (skin disease).	• Liver, • Groundnut meal sunflower, soybean meal.
Pyridoxine	Destroyed by heat.	• Participates in amino acid metabolism. • Role in 'active transport across the cell – membranes'.	• In farm animals: Anaemia, convulsions (violent contraction of muscles). • In chicks: Dermatitis.	• Liver, • Yeast, • Molasses, • Pulses.
Lipoic acid	Associated with Thiamine.	• Role in oxidative decarboxylation of pyruvic acid. • Helps in the activation of amino acids.	• No deficiency.	• Liver.
Pantothenic acid	Structural component of Co – enzyme A.	• Important in the formation of acetyl Co – A. • In combination with two – carbon fragments from carbohydrate, fat, some amino acids, enters TCA cycle.	• In farm animals: Growth goes down, lesions (wounds) in GIT and nervous tissues. • In chicks: Dermatitis.	• Alpha – alpha • Yeast, molasses, • Rice, wheat brans.
Biotin	A Co - enzyme	• Important for incorporation (addition) of one – carbon (through CO_2) into organic compounds.	• In farm animals: Weight loss, • In poultry: Dermatitis.	• Liver • Yeast • Cereals.

Folic acid	It contains Para amino benzoic acid (PABA).	• Very important in one – carbon metabolism, eg. Active CH_3 group transfers.	• In farm animals: Rare, But, may cause anaemia, poor growth.	• Liver, • Synthesized by microbes.
Choline	It has three methyl groups in its structure, hence donor of $-CH_3$ group.	• Necessary for synthesis of Lecithin. • Role in lipid metabolism.	• In farm animals: Growth goes down, fatty liver. • In chicks: Perosis, slipped tendons.	• Yeast, • Cereals, • Green leafy plant materials.
Inositol	Associated with Choline.	• Role in fatty acid metabolism.	• In farm animals: Alopecia (patchy hair). • In dairy cows: Lactation failure. • In chicks: Encephalomalacia. • Rickettsial disease	• Nuts, • Whole grains, • Yeast.
Para Amino Benzoic Acid (PABA)	Component of Folic acid.	• Helps for the synthesis of Folic acid. • Used in those organisms which do not have pre – formed sources of Folic acid.		• Liver, • Synthesized by microbes.
Cyano Cobalamine	Cyanide radical and cobalt are the structural component.	• Role in Glutamic acid metabolism, certain alcohols. • Helps in synthesis of nucleic acids.	• In farm animals: Growth goes down. • In cattle: Wasting sickness.	• Synthesized by microbes; • Liver (storage) • This is the only member which is **stored**.

Chapter 4

Digestion

Mixture of nutrients comprising carbohydrates, fats, proteins, minerals, vitamins and water are feed stuffs. From the intestinal wall, very few of such nutrients can pass directly to the body tissues, therefore they must be degraded down into simple compounds before they pass through the mucous membrane of the gastrointestinal tract (G.I.T.) into the blood and lymph. This degradation process is regarded as 'digestion'. Thereafter, the movement of these simple compounds through the mucous membrane of the G.I.Tract into the blood is called absorption. Metabolism is the utilization of these nutrients by the animal body and then excretion of the end products takes place from the body. The digestion of feeds is carried out by three means namely, mechanical action: mastication in the mouth and the muscular contraction of G.I.Tract; chemical action: this is carried out by enzymes secreted by digestive juices and microbial action: this is also enzymatic action, but the enzymes are secreted by microbes instead of host.

In ruminants, it is the rumen which harbours bacteria, protozoa and fungi (Fig. 1) ; whereas in non-ruminants, it is the large intestine (Fig. 2). There are four compartments in the stomach-reticulum, omasum, rumen and abomasums. Reticulum provides ruminant additional space for storage. Also, if by any chance, foreign bodies like nails, wires etc. reach over here alongwith feed, they are retained for longer periods and thus, soft organs are protected. Omasum squeezes out water from the feed with the help of its strong muscular walls. In the suckling calves or lambs, the two compartments-rumen and its continuation reticulum are less developed and both are joined by a tube like structure - oesophageal or reticular groove, which directly opens into abomasum. That is why in these sucklings, milk reaches straight into the abomasum, which is the true stomach. Rumen develops at about six weeks of age in these young ones. As these sucklings begin to eat solid feed, both rumen and reticulum enlarge greatly and separate. Now oesophageal or reticular groove does not exist.

Six activities take place starting from mouth to rumen - prehension, masticatin, salivation, rumination, regurgitation and eructation. In **prehension**, feed gathering takes place, which is assisted by rough tongue and teeth; In **mastication** preliminary chewing of feed is carried out by teeth; During **salivation** saliva gets mixed up with the feed not only in rumen but also in mouth and thereafter, feed is swallowed into the rumen. Enormous amounts of saliva (about 100-200 litres per day) is produced in an adult bovine and gets mixed up with the feed. Saliva makes the feed slippery and moistened. It has buffering capacity due to sodium and potassium salts of phosphate and bicarbonate. Saliva provides non protein nitrogen-urea to rumen microbes. It also exhibits anti-frothing action, because certain plants [eg. Clover (berseem)] due to presence of saponin, produce lot of froth bubbles, which get trapped in the saliva during rumination. Fermentative digestion or microbial digestion takes place in rumen, where the feed stays for longer period. The rumen capacity to hold the feed, slow passage of ingesta, continuous removal of the solubles are favourable for microbial population. Rumen is like a fermentation tank, where the feed is diluted with lot of saliva. Rumen contents contain 85 % water in two phases-lower liquid phase has suspended finer feed particles and upper dry phase is made up of coarser solid material. The feed is broken down by physical and microbial actions. During physical action, rumen contents are continuously mixed by the rhythmic contractions of its walls, which have many folds of different sizes, which are positioned in different angles to facilitate churning process. Microbial action is essentially carried out by enzymes secreted by rumen bacteria (rumen flora) and protozoa (rumen fauna). There are 10^{9-10} bacteria per milliliter of rumen fluid and they are grouped according to feed component they digest, eg. Cellulolysis is carried out by cellulolytic bacteria, proteolysis takes place by proteolytic bacteria and likewise. The number and type of bacteria, which dominate in the rumen at a particular time depend on the nature of diet. Protozoa numbering 10^6 per milliliter of rumen fluid have oligotricchs (cellulose digesters) and holotricchs (other carbohydrates digesters) in the rumen.

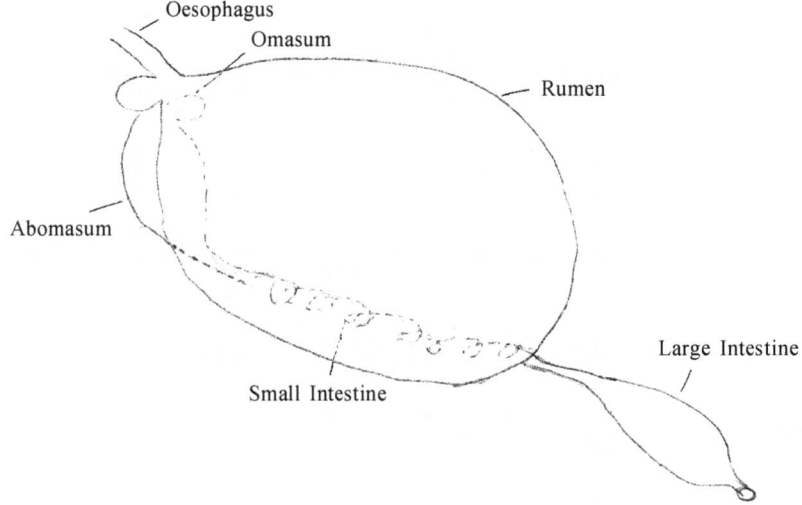

Fig. 1 : Alimentary Canal Of Ruminant [Diagrammatic Representation]

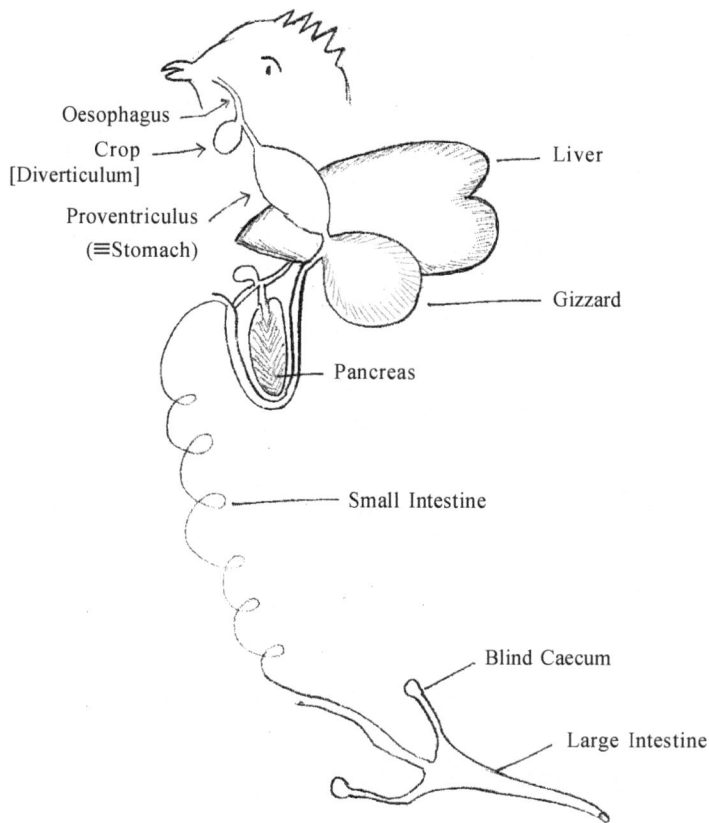

Fig. 2 : Chicken Alimentary Canal [Diagrammatic Representation]

Regurgitation is analogous to vomiting in humans. During rumination, partially fermented feed (cud) at the anterior end of rumen is drawn back into the oesophagus and returned by a reverse wave of contraction to the mouth. Any liquid is swallowed back rapidly again to rumen, but coarser material is thoroughly chewed in the mouth and then returned to rumen. The regurgitated feed is chewed 40-50 times and thus receives a much more thorough mastication than during preliminary chewing. In this way, re-mastication, re-salivation, re-rumination take place for this regurgitated digesta. Rumen conditions happen to be very suitable for microbial population – completely anaerobic (i.e. no oxygen at all, even if any trace of oxygen reaches, it would get utilized very rapidly); temperature of 39°C and a pH between 5.5 to 6.5 which is well maintained by buffering action as well as rapid absorption of volatile fatty acids (V.F.A.s) from the rumen walls. There are three functions of rumen microbes-they break down cellulose, hemicellulose to V.F.A.s, which are the primary source of energy for the host animal; they synthesize the amino acids for the synthesis of their own body coat proteins. They also synthesize vitamin 'B' complex as well as vitamin K. During **eructation** (analogous to belching in humans), methane and carbon dioxide are removed out through the mouth. Partially fermented digesta and dead microbial cells reach the abomasum (true stomach) for further digestion similar to non – ruminant, with the help of enzymes secreted by host animals. Thereafter, products are assimilated.

How ruman might have been evolved!!!

Just like **Lamarck's theory** of evolution for giraffe's long neck, it is presumed that about many thousands and thousands of years back, these ruminant animals lived in the forests and had developed an unusual habbit of eating. They used to grab the feed and swallow quickly as much as possible and then run to a safe place for protection from the wild carnivores. Later on, at leisure, they used to bring back small quantities of feed to mouth and chew it thoroughly. *Probably, that is how they might have evolved rumen over a period of time.*

Chapter 5

Digestibility Determination of Feeds

Thousands and thousands of samples of various feeds and fodders were subjected to Weende analysis for their chemical composition have been depicted in various manuals. Such proximate principles of these feeds provide only the potential value for reference or consultation purpose, but not the actual value of feedstuffs. Losses of nutrients in faeces (solids), urine (liquid), gases etc. during the digestion, absorption and metabolism of the animal should also be taken into consideration. Therefore, a need arises to conduct digestibility trial or experiment for the feeds in the ruminant animals. Major portion of the nutrients present in the feeds are not properly digested in the gastrointestinal tract (G.I.T.), hence not completely available to the animal body. Digestibility is that portion of a feed or any single nutrient of feed, which is not excreted in the faeces or dung and it is therefore, assumed to be absorbed by the animal. When this digestibility is expressed in percentage, it is termed as 'digestibility coefficient (D.C.)'.

$$\text{Digestibility coefficient} = \frac{\text{Kgs of dry matter feed eaten - kgs of dry matter in faeces}}{\text{Kgs of dry matter feed eaten}} \times 100$$

Digestibility is calculated for dry matter, crude protein, crude fibre, ether extract and nitrogen – free extract, but not for 'ash' content because it does not contribute energy and moreover, gastric secretions (eg. Pancreatic, bile juices etc.) add into more minerals in the digesta. If a cow is eating daily twenty kgs of fresh green maize with twenty five percent dry matter and excreting two kgs of dry matter in the faeces, that means five minus two, equalling to three kgs of feed, which might have been digested hence, 0.60 is the digestibility. When this is expressed in percentage, that is sixty percent, it would be digestibility coefficient of green maize in question.

For the **"measurement of digestibility of fodder"**, at least six healthy ruminant adult animals of same species, age and gender are taken. This is just to avoid animal to animal variation for digestibility. Generally male animals are taken to facilitate easy collection of faeces or dung samples from these animals. The animals are fed on fodder to be probed for at least three weeks to remove any effect of previous feed and also, that makes the animals adaptable or familiar to this new feed. This period is called adaptation or pre-experimental period.

Thereafter the actual experimental period of eight days starts. During this trial period, the animals are kept in separate stalls or partitions (poultry birds in different pens or cages), so that their faeces or excreta may not mix up with each other. During this experimental or collection period, daily record of feed offered, residual feed left and faeces voided are made on twenty hour basis. The representative samples of these three types of feed are carried to laboratory daily and kept in hot air oven for complete drying. After drying, these samples are dropped in the big, **environmental friendly poly bags** daily, so that at the end of the experimental period, the entire daily collected samples may be pooled together for the proximate analysis later. This method is applicable for such feeds which are fed alone and supply bulk for the 'rumen–fill, for example green maize, oat, grasses, legumes etc.

Indirect determination of digestibility or difference method is carried out for certain feeds, which can not be fed alone and hence their digestibility coefficient can not be measured directly, for example concentrate feeds-cereal grains, oil seed cakes, by-products of cereals, because they do not supply the 'bulk'. Therefore in this indirect system of digestibility determination, two digestibility trials are undertaken. In the first trial, the digestibility of nutrients is determined by feeding a 'basal maintenance type of fodder' but without the 'test' concentrate feed. In the second trial, fodder of first trial and test concentrate feed are fed together and thereafter, difference of both trials is accounted. Here it will be assumed that the digestibility coefficients of nutrients in the fodder obtained from the first trial will remain the same in the second trial. Hence the total nutrients voided in the faeces from the portion belonging to the fodder of first trial is subtracted from that of second trial. The remaining faecal nutrients are considered to have come from the 'test' feed.

Chapter 6

Expressing the Energy Value of Feeds

There are three types of systems for expressing the energy value of feeds and many examples have been depicted in each of these systems the world over but here, one example has been taken up in each of these categories.

Digestible Nutrient Type

For example, Total digestible nutrients (TDN) system: Digestibility coefficients of various organic nutrients like carbohydrate, fat and protein are determined by digestibility trials, which can be utilized to be involved for total digestible nutrients as a measure of nutritive value of feeds. Here only faecal enegy loss has been considered barring losses from other channels. Hence roughages are overestimated by such calculations. Otherwise, this method is simple, economical and has some basis for animals to be fed on such standard in India. The TDN value is expressed in percentage as following :

% TDN = % dig. C.P. + % dig. C.F. + % dig. N.F.E. + [% dig. E.E. X 2.25]

where,

Dig.	= Digestible
C.P.	= Crude Protein
C.F.	= Crude Fibre
E.E.	= Ether Extract
N.F.E.	= 100 - [C.P.% + E.E.% + C.F.% + Ash%] on dry matter basis

TDN content of any feed represents energy of calorific value of that particular feed. The digestibility of crude protein is included in this equation because of the fact that, excess of protein eaten by the animals, serves as a source of energy to the body. Merit of this system is that, TDN of a feed can be easily determined and demerit or limitation being – unless the dry matter of a feed is digestible, it can have no TDN value. For example, lignin has a very high gross energy or calorific value but it can not be digested by ruminants. Hence, lignin has no TDN value.

Production value type

For example, Starch Equivalent or S.E. system originated from Germany, hence followed in those areas of Europe and takes into account almost all the losses involved in digestion of feed. The method is based on carbon – nitrogen balance studies without the help of any costly equipment but faced some criticism too. The animals were kept in big animal calorimeter, where different sources of energy-losses could be determined to the best of their ability. When it was ensured that the ration on which the animals were neither gaining nor losing weight (by measuring the intake and outgo of both carbon and nitrogen) then pure starch, straw pulp that is cellulose, wheat gluten (protein) and oil were added to this diet and determined the carbon and nitrogen separately again. Feeds for productive purposes are measured in terms of starch values.

$$S.E. = \frac{\text{Weight of fat stored / unit of feed}}{\text{Weight of fat stored / unit of starch}} \times 100$$

That is, amount of feed required to produce as much animal fat as is being produced by unit amount of starch, when fed in addition to maintenance. For example, if linseed cake has got SE of 75, which means that hundred kgs of linseed cake can produce as much fat as 75 kgs of pure starch when fed in addition to maintenance ration.

Comparative type

For example, Scandinavian system, which is followed in Denmark, Sweden, Norway, Iceland etc. This system is based purely on practical method of feeding, where the comparative production of growth, work, fattening are ascertained by means of group feeding experiments. Similar type of animals are selected with respect to age, weight and productive capacity and are placed on adaptation period with a standard diet so that animals may react similarly to achieve uniformity. For the experimental period, separate test feeds are included in each group along with a basal ration. One kg of barley (or corn or wheat) is used as a "feed unit" instead of starch, which was used as a unit in starch – equivalent system. In practice, comparative feed values are applicable on the basis of actual result and hence any specific value of feed received proper recognition, in addition to its protein and energy value. Due to diversified farming as well as the grains were of different types in different countries, the feed units also differed. Hence, the system was not applicable in other countries including Asia.

Chapter 7

Partition of Energy

The animal body can be imagined as a machine, which is getting input of desired or available feed given by the farmer and this animal body after processing through various metabolic activities, output of product is given off. Feed is composed of organic nutrients-carbohydrate, fat and protein and after reaching in the animal body, used for constructive work, for example synthesis of body tissues and other associated work. Later, milk or egg is produced as an output. Now putting the same perspective in terms of energy, that is, these organic nutrients of the feed contain chemical energy and after reaching in the animal body, used as mechanical energy in muscles or heat energy in metabolism. The energy in the body would be utilized for the synthesis of body tissues or other productive output, for example, draft work by bullocks. Therefore, energy is primarily required for the maintenance of the body and then, for the productive purposes :

- Growth for all the farm animals
- Milk from cow, buffalo, sheep, goat
- Eggs from poultry, duck, turkey
- Wool from sheep
- Meat from fattening animals under the law, for example – mutton, chevon, pork, chicken.

[Beef is produced in Western or Gulf Countries under their culture]

Partition of gross energy is depicted in the flow chart diagram. 'Gross energy' is the quantity of heat produced by the complete oxidation of unit weight of feed. This is measured by bomb calorimeter. In this way hundred per cent calorific value of any nutrient or feed would be obtained. 'Digestive energy' is achieved after the loss of faecal energy is taken into account. This is the first source of loss (about 30%) which is measured by digestibility trial and thus, on an average about seventy per cent would be digestible energy of the total. After further losses (about 10%) of urinary and methane energy have been considered, 'metabolisable energy' is witnessed, which would be on an average sixty per cent of the total. Urinary energy is observed in the nitrogen containing substances-urea, hippuric acid, allantoin and can be measured in digestibility trial, whereas methane by respiration chamber or face mask method. Thus, the energy is lost as chemical energy through solid (faeces), liquid (urine) and gas (methane); but energy is lost as heat also, called 'heat increment'. Because of inefficiency of energetic reactions of animal body as well as different processes of rumen digestion (mastication, propulsion of feed along alimentary canal, regurgitation, fermentation by microbes etc.), heat increment results. The balance about fourty per cent, accounts for the 'net energy', which is actually available to the animal for useful purposes. Again, it may further be partitioned to 'net energy for maintenance' utilized for the vital physiological functions and leaves the body as heat. This heat together with heat increment is the 'total heat production'. Another part is 'net energy for production' or 'energy-retention', which is used for productive purposes, like growth, milk yield, wool, meat production etc. This may be measured by carbon-nitrogen balance experiment. The flow chart of partitioning of energy with losses has been depicted in the Flow chart 2.

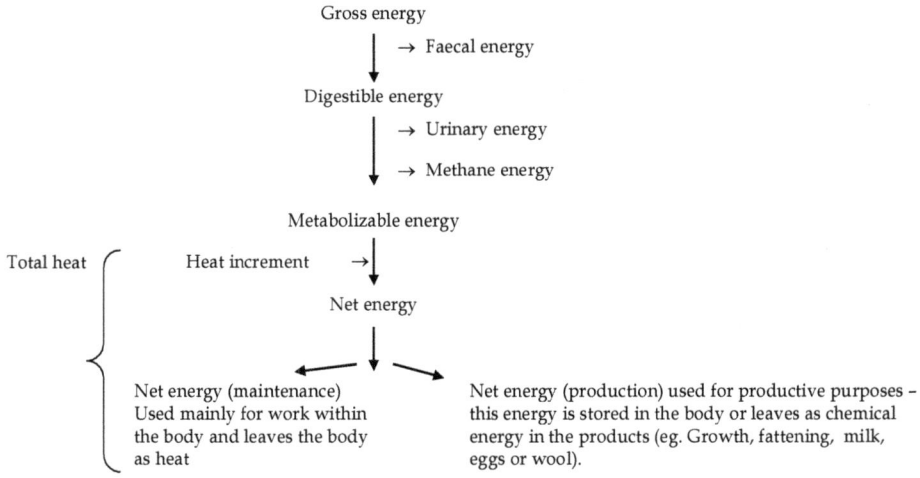

Flow chart 2: Partitioning of gross energy

Chapter 8

Expressing the Protein Value of Feeds

Crude protein of feeds contain true protein and non-protein nitrogen. True protein is made up amino acids and for the maximum efficiency, feed must have essential amino acids in correct proportion, correct balance as well as non essential amino acids should also be in sufficient amounts. About digestion in simple stomached animals, the true protein is degraded to oligo peptides (less than ten peptides) in the stomach, subsequently to mono peptide and amino acids in the small intestine. Thereafter amino acids are assimilated in the small intestine. But in ruminants, the situation is complex in the sense that feed proteins get digested in the rumen but even amino acids are also broken down by microbes and thereafter, amino and carboxylic groups are released. Secondly, synthesis of new amino acids or proteins takes place for the formation of their own microbial body coat. Because of these reasons, the approach for protein evaluation or expression is different in ruminant and non-ruminant animal. Further, non-protein nitrogen portion of feed can not be utilized effectively by non – ruminants like swine and poultry. These animals are usually fed with oil cakes, cereals and cereal by-products, which are poor in non-protein nitrogen compounds, however, young succulent fodders, clover etc. are rich in such compounds.

In the laboratory, crude protein may estimated by kjeldahl's method and true protein may be precipitated from non protein nitrogen fraction by treating with cupric hydroxide or trichloro acetic acid. The precipitate is filtered off and subjected to kjeldahl's process. For experimental evaluation of non ruminants – albino or wistar rats, rabbits, guinea pigs or poultry birds are taken. Casein (milk protein) or albumen (egg protein) are fed to these animals as reference or standard to be compared with the test protein for a period of four weeks and any of the following methods are undertaken to look for the protein quality based on response of animals.

Nitrogen balance experiment : Here, nitrogen consumed, nitrogen excreted in excreta as well as in eggs or milk are considered.

When, in an animal,
- N intake = N output, it is said to be N equilibrium
- N intake > N output, it is said to be + ve N equilibrium
- N intake < N output, it is said to be − ve N equilibrium

Protein Efficiency Ratio (PER): Here growth of the albino rat is measured in terms of weight gain per unit weight of protein eaten.

$$\text{P.E.R.} = \frac{\text{Gain in body weight (gms)}}{\text{Protein consumed (gms)}}$$

Protein Replacement Value (PRV): This method measures as to how much quantity of 'test protein' is equivalent to standard protein, that is, how much quantity of test protein can replace a standard protein. For this to achieve, two nitrogen balance experiments are conducted – one for standard protein of high quality, for example, egg or milk protein and second for the test protein.

$$\text{P.R.V.} = \frac{A - B}{N \text{ intake}} \quad [\text{where, } A = N \text{ balance of standard protein};\ B = N \text{ balance of test protein}]$$

Biological Value (B.V.): This the percentage of nitrogen absorbed, which is actually retained by the animal. For this to obtain, a nitrogen balance experiment is conducted. Recordings are taken for nitrogen intake, nitrogen excreted in faeces and urine.

$$\text{B.V.} = \frac{\text{Nitrogen intake} - [\text{Faecal N} + \text{Urinary N}]}{\text{Nitrogen intake} - \text{Faecal nitrogen}} \times 100$$

Faecal nitrogen also contains some nitrogen of metabolic origin, that is 'metabolic faecal nitrogen (MFN)' and similarly, urinary nitrogen has nitrogen from metabolic origin, that is 'endogenous urinary nitrogen (EUN)'. Therefore, in another set of trial, animals are given nitrogen-free diet and then compared with the experimental animals. Faecal nitrogen minus metabolic faecal nitrogen in place of faecal nitrogen as well as urinary nitrogen minus endogenous urinary nitrogen in place of urinary nitrogen are replaced in the above formula to get the correct picture.

For **ruminant animals**, most common way of expression is the digestible crude protein (D.C.P.) values, which are calculated with the help of literature values of corresponding digestibility co-efficient in some countries including in India.

Hence,

D.C.P. % = C.P. % X Digestibility coefficient.

There is lot of variation for the roughages compared to concentrates; therefore, regression equation is suggested in some countries :

D.C.P. % = [C.P. % X 0.9] – 3.7

Protein Equivalent (P.E.): This is followed in some European countries.

$$P.E. = \frac{\% \text{ D.C.P.} + \% \text{ digestible true protein}}{2}$$

[Here, equivalent is being used in place of D.C.P. Non – protein nitrogen fraction is given half the nutritive value of the true protein].

Partition of Feed Nitrogen :

The newer system of protein evaluation in ruminants is based on the partition of feed nitrogen in Rumen Degradable Nitrogen and Undegradable Nitrogen. It has been observed that Undegradable Nitrogen or Bypass Nitrogen is not completely absorbed from the intestinal tract and further partitioned into :

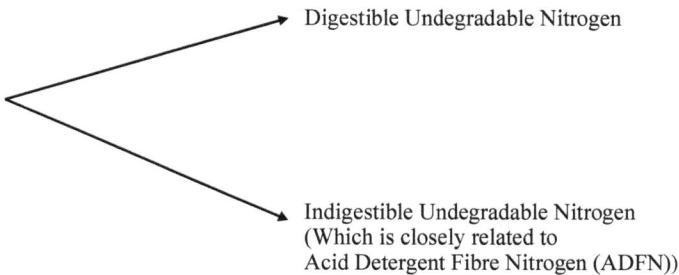
Digestible Undegradable Nitrogen

Indigestible Undegradable Nitrogen
(Which is closely related to
Acid Detergent Fibre Nitrogen (ADFN))

Chapter 9

Feeding Standards

Declaration of facts about the amounts of nutrients required by the various classes of livestock for different physiological functions like maintenance, growth, lactation, egg production, wool production etc. are in general termed as "Feeding standards". **Nutrient requirement** is the statement of what animals on an average require for a particular function. **Allowance** is greater than the required amount by a 'safety margin' which is allowed for variations in requirement between individual animals. Such standards may be expressed in quantities or in dietary proportions, for example **gram per day,** this method of expression is used mainly for animals given exact quantities of feeds; or **gram per kilogram of the diet**, this method is used for animals fed to appetite.

Various units are used for feeding standards – for ruminants, the energy requirements may be stated in terms of net energy, metabolizable energy or feed units and protein requirements in terms of crude protein, digestible crude protein or metabolizable protein. It is obviously desirable that the units used in the standards should be the same as those used in the evaluation of feeds. For dairy cows, the requirements are given separately for maintenance and for milk production. But for growing chickens, they are given for maintenance and growth combined. In some instances, the requirements for single functions are not known, for example, vitamins and trace elements. As mentioned above, in feeding practice, the requirement amount is accompanied by the addition of a 'safety factor'.

Justification of 'Safety factor'

There may be some range for the requirement of any nutrient in the individual animals with some mean value (say X). Much of the variation will undoubtedly reflect real difference between animals; however some of the variation may be caused by inaccuracies in the methods of measurement used. With this variation, if above mean of X is applied in practice, then :

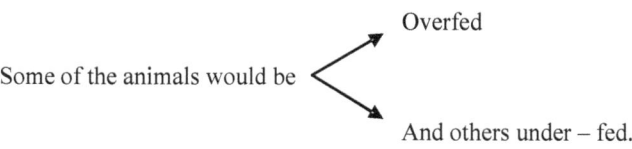

Underfeeding would be considered as the great offence. The above 'safety margin' of X would ensure that no animals would be underfed. But still, there may be some exceptions, which may have higher requirements. If this happens to be capricious addition, then they devised a better method based **mathematically** on the expected variation between animals. This would mean that the animals with larger variation should cover with the greater 'safety factor'.

Safety factors have been criticized

Such criticism occurred on the following grounds :
- a) **Over-feeding :** It is wasteful procedure, because maximum of the population to ensure that the remaining are not grossly underfed. For some nutrients, they are justifiable for which, cost of over-supply is relatively low, for example magnesium. Their deficiency may cause severe disorders and even death.
- b) **Over-supply of nutrients :** For those nutrients which supply energy, safety margins may not be justified. Because, over-feeding of energy is expected to be costly and then secondly, animals might store excessive amounts of fat, which may not be desirable (however they may respond to excess in terms of increase in rate of production which may not be desirable).

We may agree that 'variations' do occur between 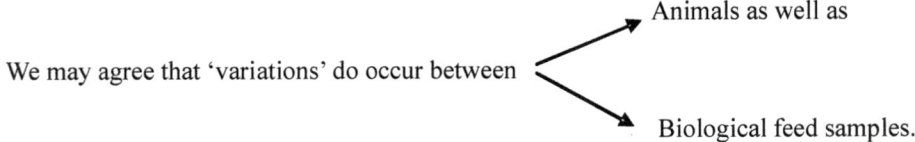 Animals as well as Biological feed samples.

The art of stockman in the finer adjustments can not be neglected

Obviously, then there would be **'inaccuracies'** in the above, which may invariably be attended while applying feeding standards. For this reason, the feeding standards should be considered as guides to feeding practice. After all, such rules (which should be **'flexible'**) would not replace "the art of the stockman".

The feeding standards are just guides

These are designed to be the general references for practice but should be considered subject to modifications in the light of the following :
- a) Economic factors to be taken into account.

Feeding Standards

b) Therefore, modifications may be called for "in the interest of" obtaining the rate of gain or level of production that seems the most economical in terms of current feed costs and market price of the product.

c) No standard can be complete guide to feeding because other factors such as – palatability and physical nature of the ration must also be taken into account.

Following are some standards which are available for feeding the various categories of livestock in different countries :

1. **Agricultural Research Council (A.R.C.)** : Research scientists had drawn up feeding standards in England under this council. The **Technical Committee on Responses to Nutrients** had taken up responsibility in 1983 for both revising standards and producing practical manuals and subsequently Commonwealth Agricultural Bureau had published reports [ARC (1981, 1984)].

2. **National Research Council (NRC)** : A statement of quantitative needs for all the recognized nutrients for farm animals was undertaken by the **Committee on Animal Nutrition** of above council in 1942. For reviewing the literature, sub-committees of experts for each class of stock were accordingly set up. "Recommended Nutrient Allowances" for farm animals, comprising separate reports by each class of stock were published in the beginning of 1944 [Committee on Animal Nutrition (1949, 1953, 1954, 1957, 1958, 1960)]. Following the lead of the NRC Food and Nutrition Board, the term **"allowance"** was first adopted for use in **human dietary standards**. In general, these allowances were set higher than average determined requirements to provide a "margin of safety". The Committee on Animal Nutrition decided to set forth intakes considered adequate for normal growth, health and production, based on the average needs of groups of animals to achieve these results (and not to include such margins in future recommendations). Therefore, it was agreed that future reports would be designated as "nutrient requirements", instead of 'recommended nutrient allowances'. The pooled judgment of a group of experts in the field of the species in question, submitted their reports to NRC. These NRC reports should be considered the most authoritative statements of the nutritional needs of farm animals at least for feeding practice in United States of America.

3. **Indian Standards:** Based on the mid Morrison standards for feeding cattle, Ray, Sen and Ranjhan (1978) standards for Zebu cattle and buffaloes have been given. In 1991, Ranjhan had further revised the above and then standards for poultry were also included. On the basis of extensive research

carried out in India since 1960, these standards were chalked out for feeding animals under Indian conditions. Indian Council of Agricultural Research has also given nutrient requirements for cattle and poultry.

[These days "Burean of Indian standards (B.I.S.)" are available].

Chapter 10

Fasting Heat Production

Maintenance
When an animal is being fed for growth, fattening, milk secretion or other productive function, a considerable part of its feed is utilized for supporting body processes which are vital, irrespective of new tissue or product is being formed. This demand for feed is referred to as the "Maintenance requirement"; because it includes the amount needed to keep intact the tissues of animal which is not growing, working or yielding any product. There would be tissue break down with the accompanying loss in weight, leading to undesirable consequences, provided such need for feed is not met.

The fasting catabolism
The fasting animal doing no external work and not producing in any way is still carrying on a variety of internal physiological processes, which are absolutely vital for life. Obviously the nutrients required to support these internal activities must come from the break down of body tissue itself. This destruction of body tissue is termed as the "Fasting catabolism" and this can be measured in terms of the waste products discarded through the various paths of excretion.

Energy catabolism of fasting
The energy expended in the fasting animal is converted into heat, which can be measured in direct or indirect calorimeter. For measuring fasting catabolism at its minimum value, it becomes imperative to eliminate all the influences leading to increase heat production above the minimum expenditure compatible with the maintenance of life in so far as possible. Such a minimum value is called "Basal-metabolism" or BMR. The conditions essential for a true minimum value of fasting catabolism can most nearly be attained in human being are specified as following :
1. Good nutritive condition
2. Environmental temperature of $25°C$ [$77°F$]
3. Relaxing on reclining couch prior to and during study
4. Post–absorptive state.

A good nutrition condition implies that the previous diet was adequate in energy and protein; otherwise a poor state of nutrition tends to decrease the heat production during fasting. The environmental temperature is specified to assume that no tissue break down is occurring to keep up the temperature of the body above critical as well as there is no start of fever which may increase heat production below the hyper thermal rise. Both of the above two conditions are entirely realizable in the animals. But it is much less subject control the minimum muscular activity in farm animals as per the third condition. This is due to miscellaneous movements of the animal may be expected to spend a variable portion of the experimental period standing and lying down. However, **horse** is an exception, because of the structure of its ligaments, seems to rest as comfortably standing as lying, without any increased energy expenditure. The post absorptive state is easy in all except in ruminants, where 3-4 days fasting is required to ensure minimum methane (CH_4) excretion as well as little or no carbohydrate is being burnt after fasting. The latter situation is characterized by the non–protein respiratory quotient of fat (RQ of 0.707) is frequently referred to as basal metabolism.

Resting metabolism

This term denotes the heat eliminated when an animal is lying at rest, though not strictly in thermo-neutral environment or in the post absorptive state.

$W^{0.75}$

At an early stage in the study of basal metabolism, it was recognized that fasting heat production was more nearly proportional to the surface area and it became customary to compare values for animals of different sizes by expressing them in relation to surface area. Rubner developed a concept: Surface–area law, that the heat given off by all warm-blooded animals is as following.

Fasting heat production ∝ Body surface area

In view of the difficulties and uncertainties involved in measuring surface area, formulae were devised for computing it from body weight, recognizing that :

Surface ∝ to some fractional power of weight

The above surface-area theory rested primarily on the knowledge derived from investigation and that it does not have so general an application as previously thought. While the concept has been and still remains very useful, it is agreed that the previous methods of measuring or estimating surface area give such variable results that a statement of heat elimination per unit of surface had a very limited meaning except in terms of the specific method used in obtaining the surface measure. The body surface is not a constant but varies with the position of the body. The fact that the skin is **elastic** causes its measurement to vary with conditions :

a) Whether measured on the live animal, or
b) After its removal.

The surface area of animals is obviously difficult to measure and methods were therefore, devised for predicting it from their body weight. The basis for such methods is that, in bodies of the same shape and of equal density,

Surface area $\propto$ to the 2/3rd power of weight

The logical development of this approach was to omit the calculation of surface area and express fasting metabolism in relation to $W^{0.67}$. By now, it became practice among investigators of energy – metabolism of animals to use a fractional or decimal power of weight instead of surface area, as the unit of reference.

On the basis of an analysis of a very large number of basal metabolism data of mature animals of different species ranging :

From mice (0.02 kg) to elephants (4000 kgs);

Brody suggested the power 0.73. A link between fasting metabolism and body weight was examined further; it was found that the closest relationship was between -

Metabolism and $W^{0.73}$ (and not $W^{0.67}$)

The function $W^{0.73}$ was used as a reference base for fasting metabolism for farm animals until 1964. Brody later eliminated the second decimal, because it was giving a false idea of the precision involved and thus, adopted the power **0.7**. This general field had also been extensively studied and reviewed by Kliber (1947) who felt that $W^{¾}$ provided a better-fitting formula for relating basal metabolism to body size than does $W^{0.7}$. It was a rounded off exponent to 0.75. There has been considerable discussion whether surface area or $W^{0.75}$ (often called **Metabolic live weight**) was better base. Mathematically there is nothing to choose between the two bases, because, their relationships with fasting metabolism were equally close.

Both are in use. The ¾th power has the practical advantage of being readily calculated by the use of a **slide rule** or by **arithmetic**. While the other requires the use of **logarithms**. The basal metabolism per day for adult homeotherms may be represented by the general formula :

Basal metabolism (kcal / day) = 70 $W^{0.75}$

[Where W is weight in kgs, the coefficient 70 represents an average value for the kilo calories of basal heat produced per unit of metabolic size in experiments with groups of adult animals.]

The unit of reference for metabolic size $W^{0.7}$ or $W^{3/4}$, is useful as a base value for calculating energy requirement for various purposes and for measuring feed-efficiency. In such use, it should be kept in mind that the unit is an average value subject to variability according to individuals and species. Brody noted for example that, in the data which he analyzed the power of weight found for mature birds of different species ranged from 0.62 to 0.70. For dogs of different sizes, the average was 0.6 and for rabbits 0.82.

Energy requirements

- When, energy intake is Zero [i.e. Animal is fasted]; then, there will be energy loss from animal body, Negative energy balance. [That means animal is using its body reserves – glycogen from liver and depot fat from adipose tissue to provide energy for maintaining its most vital physiological functions – blood circulation, heart beating, breathing from lungs, kidney and brain function etc.]
- When, energy intake is increased a little [i.e. some feed is given]; then, energy loss from body diminishes or reduced to some extent.
- When, energy intake is increased to such a level or extent that, energy loss is minimum or say Zero. [That means, this is the minimum quantity of feed, which must be given to the animal, so that the animal experiences neither net gain nor loss of that nutrient and this is the **'maintenance level or requirement for energy'**.
- Now, if energy intake is further increased; then, energy retention or storing will start in the animal – either in its body tissues (adipose) or in its products.

Protein requirements

It has been observed that there are following three types of nitrogen losses –

a) Faecal : nitrogen (that is, undigested nitrogen of feed origin) + Metabolic faecal nitrogen [**M.F.N.** from body origin, for example – enzymes, dead microbes (body coat proteins), aberrated cell residues of epithelial lining coming from alimentary canal].

b) Urinary : nitrogen (of feed origin, urea or nitrogen containing compounds coming from amino acid or protein catabolism; allantoin in birds) + Endogenous urinary nitrogen [**E.U.N.** from creatine of muscles].

c) Small dermal losses: (a) Scurf: scales of skin epidermis; (b) Keratinized tissue: hair, nails, horn etc.

Following are experimental situations to probe the protein requirement:

1. If an animal is placed on a nitrogen - free diet (but sufficient in energy), then nitrogen loss still occurs through urine excretion. [This nitrogen loss represents that portion of nitrogen, which could not be re-used in the body].

2. On the nitrogen – free diet, the nitrogen falls for several days in the urine and then stabilizes to a minimum constant level, which is maintained from the **point a** in the graph shown. Therefore, this minimum nitrogen – loss is the 'Maintenance level of protein'. Now there are two sub-situations:

   a) If **sufficient** energy is available to animal, then the minimum level stabilizes.

   b) If the energy level is **not sufficient**, then there will be further loss of nitrogen in urine from the **point b** in the graph shown.

3. When nitrogen is re-introduced, then nitrogen level starts restoring.

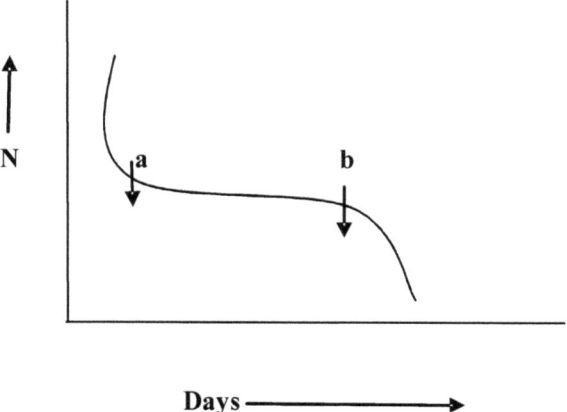

Graph 1: Nitrogen level goes down in the urine.

Chapter 11

Animal Growth and Nutrition

The increase in size and weight of farm animals is the simplest manifestation. The life in the animals begins with a single cell weighing practically nothing, then grow to reach mature weights ranging from 1 kg to 800 kg or more for a bison. From conception to maturity, animals growth can be depicted by a sigmoid (S-shaped) graph :

- Foetal period
- Birth to puberty

  } there is an acceleration of growth

- After puberty to
- Just prior to maturity

  } there is deceleration of growth and reaches a very low value

Practically there may be deviation from above pattern due to environmental and nutritional features. Retardation of growth may be observed due to feed scarcity during cold or dry seasons. Vice-versa will happen when there is feed abundance. **Intensive husbandry** generally follows sigmoid growth of animals. Whereas, idealized pattern of growth would be deviated in the growth rate of animals, when reared under natural (**extensive**) conditions; exhibiting interrupted curves. While growing, **development** of various parts of the animal, defined as anatomical components (for example legs), as organs (for example liver) or as tissues (for example muscle) grow at different rates. By the time of maturity, the proportions of the animal changes. For example in cattle:

- At birth: Head is relatively large, 6.2 % of the body weight.
- At body weight of 100 kg: Head is 4.5 % of body weight.
- At further maturity: continues to decline.

Sir John Hammond of Cambride University opined for the development of farm animals as a series of **"growth waves"**. For example, major tissues of the animal body:

- Early life (including pre – birth life): Grow rapidly, because nerve and bone tissues have priority for available nutrients,
- Later: Muscle has priority and
- Finally: Adipose tissue grows most rapidly.

Growth waves would be overlapping during rapid early growing period, because animals start forming substantial fat depots during early stages of life, while the progress still continues for muscle growth. There is a pretty well interaction between animal growth and nutrition and each can influence the other. The nutrient requirements are determined by growth pattern and vice – versa is also true. Also, in such interaction, composition of product of growth for example meat is also determined by growth pattern. Therefore, animal growth and development may be modified by control of nutrition.

- **When animals are raised for meat production:** The farmer generally aims to produce carcasses that would meet a particular specifications for weight and composition.
- **When animals are raised for breeding or lactation or egg production:** Then farmer follows different patterns other than meat animals.

How growth can be controlled by nutrition !!!

Generally, there are two fold aims of any farmer or scientist for controlling animal growth by nutrition:

- To achieve a high growth – rate by using the nutritional resources.
- To fulfill the demand of consumer by producing a carcass that meets such requirement.

Animal's nutrient intake, particularly energy, is controlled by its growth – rate, energy is considered to be the **"pace maker"** of animal production. Hence, influenced by both natural change (for example climate) and imposed change in the animal's energy supply would be reflected in its rate of growth. For reducing the 'overhead' cost of maintenance per unit of meat – production, a rapid rate of growth is desirable.

- In developed countries: Animal feeds are readily available for the animal production industries, although their use may be restricted by cost.
- In many developing countries: Inadequate supplies are being spread over too many animals due to small or non – existent supplies of feeds, particularly of high energy concentrates.

Fat was a highly prized component of meat in the past. Before, twentieth century, there was shortage of vegetable oils, and to fuel their manual work, many consumers needed a high energy intake. Hence, the people were looking for such an ideal meat-animal which fattened early in life and this was possible by 'genetic selection of small, early-maturing breeds'. The twin purposes – rapid early growth as well as a desirable carcass (that is, to have a greater amount of fat in each unit of gain), were found to be compatible with each other. But in current practice, the consumers have become very conscious of health, therefore, preferring lean-carcass (that is, fat-less). For this reason, they are avoiding the use of such breeds that are larger and late-maturing and large breed growing rapidly, would be sacrificed when relatively immature.

Another way: Repartitioning agents, for example: oestrogens, androgens, growth hormone, β-adrenergic agonist that alter the partition of energy deposition towards protein and away from fat. Growth hormone was a powerful repartitioning agent which had paved way for the use of "Genetic engineering" to increase the animals' own production of hormone. But, in most of Europe and many other countries, such practice has been banned due to 'residues' left in the meat. Therefore, nutritional approach became more acceptable method and sometimes, those two purposes may be put together: (i) maximizing lean tissue or (b) protein deposition. To achieve this, protein supply should be optimal (that is, improve protein nutrition for livestock) and also, protein supply should match energy supply. In ruminants, **energy : protein** balance is set by the rumen. Still a strategy of providing **"Rumen un – degradable protein"**, but digestible in the lower gut would be a good answer.

Therefore,
- Dietary energy deficit would be made-up by the use of body fat
- While, depositing protein at the same time.

Opportunity for nutritional control of growth
Phasing of nutrient intake

Mc Meekan of New Zealand, under the direction of Sir John Hammond at the University of Cambridge, had demonstrated – how plane of nutrition can be adjusted in relation to the growth rate of different parts to influence composition of the carcass at market weight of swine.

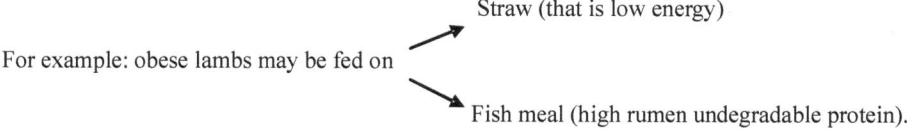

For example: obese lambs may be fed on
- Straw (that is low energy)
- Fish meal (high rumen undegradable protein).

i) **High-High:** First group of animals were kept on a high plane of nutrition throughout a slaughter weight at 180 days.

ii) **Low-Low:** This group was fed on a low plane to the same weight, 300 days being required.

iii) **High-Low:** The animals were fed high (an abundant supply of nutrients) in the early stage of swine – life, followed by low plane of nutrition (shortage of feed supply) during the later stage.

iv) **Low-High:** Received reverse rate of feeding that of (III).

The High – Low system produced the "best" – bacon type as a result of the (i) heavy feeding during the period of maximum bone and muscle formation, (ii) the limited feeding, when fat deposition normally predominates. For many years, bacon swine had their feed intake restricted so that they were fed according to such sequence in order to limit fat deposition. Sometime back, the genotype of bacon swine had been modified to provide animals that voluntarily restrict their intake as they approach bacon weight, and thus avoid excessive fat deposition. Low – High system produced a hog with characteristics of the – early maturing, lard type. Such animals with most fat and least muscle fitted the growth wave theory, as a deficiency of nutrients in early life appeared to have restricted the muscle growth that had the highest priority at that stage. Low – Low system had too large a portion of bone, poor development of loin and hind quarter and too little fat. **One school of thought** had shown that restricting the feed intake of market hogs or "diluting" highly digestible rations with fibrous feeds, during the 'finishing period', improves the carcass for bacon by reducing fat deposition and increasing the actual size of the muscle area. As expected, there was a decreased rate of gain and an increase in the length of feeding period accordingly.

Another school of thought had opined phase feeding as a term used to describe offering of several diets for a relatively short period of time in order to closely meet the swine's nutrient requirements. With current feeding strategy, it is not likely to meet the animals' nutrient requirement which rapidly changes according to their age. By phase feeding, the nutrient requirements could be met more closely and it provides a more economical and environmentally sound feeding programme for such livestock. From numerous research results, swine reared on phase feeding programme seemed to grow as well as swine reared on conventional feeding programme (usually 1 or 2 phase feeding in finishing period). However, excretion of nutrients could be dramatically reduced with phase feeding programme. Reduced amounts of nitrogen and phosphorous were reported by various researchers. To apply phase feeding into practical swine industry, digestibility or availability of ingredients, gender, genetics, growth potential, physiological status of the animals and feed additives should be carefully considered as these factors will affect the growth performance and nutrient utilization of the animals. Phase feeding can be applied more efficiently when producers have **computerized feeding system**. Thus, there might be a need to define appropriate number of phases and proper levels of nutrients supply for swine of each growth stage.

Yet another school of thought for poultry professionals suggested for **phase feeding of laying hens**, wherein phase feeding refers essentially to reductions in the protein and amino acid of the diet as the bird progresses through a laying cycle. The concept of phase feeding was based on the fact that as birds get older their feed intake increases, while their egg production decreases. For this reason, it should be economical to reduce the nutrient concentration of the diet. At this time, it is pertinent to consider a conventional egg production curve of a layer, and superimpose both egg weight and daily egg mass output. If nutrient density is to be reduced, this should not occur immediately after peak egg numbers, but rather after peak egg mass had been achieved. There were two reasons for reducing the level of dietary protein and amino acids during the later stages of egg production namely, to reduce feed costs and secondly, to reduce egg size. The advantages of the first point were readily apparent if protein costs were high, but the advantages of the second point were not so easily defined and will vary depending upon the price of eggs. When a producer was being paid a premium for extra large and jumbo eggs, there was no advantage to using a phase feeding programme unless egg shell quality was a problem.

Phenomenon of compensatory growth (in cattle)

In the ancient time or natural systems of animal production, a **low-high sequence**, that is, in early life a period of feed-shortage to a period of an abundant supply of nutrients in the later stage of life was followed. During the high phase, cattle for example, grew very rapidly. Such compensatory growth allowed them to "catch up" on animals that were not subjected to a low phase. The **cause of** compensatory growth and **effects on** body composition were variable. Compensatory animals had more nutrients available for growth, because they eat more per unit of body weight than others. Also, if they grew more in bone and muscle than fat, then :

- Less energy per unit weight would be present in their gains.
- A greater gain in live weight would be enhanced by each unit of energy intake.

Therefore in nutshell, the weight of the animal was the primary determinant of composition and hence of nutrient requirements for growth.

Chapter 12

Lactation

Biochemical and Physiological Role of Lactation is Tremendous

On a large scale, feed nutrients are converted into milk constituents by considerable biochemical and physiological processes. A high yielder of dairy may produce five times dry matter in the milk, as is present in her own body, during a single lactation. Still there are records of cows, which have produced in a year's milk over five times the organic matter of their own bodies. Certain other high yielders, which over a life time, have secreted organic matter in the milk equivalent to thirty five times that present in their own tissues. The noteworthy physiological performance is represented in the milk secretion of sow nursing a larger litter. Human organism is capable of producing an astonishing output of milk. The feed provides raw materials from which the milk constituents are derived. Some of these milk components are synthesized in the udder, for which energy is supplied again by feed. Therefore, the amount and composition of milk dictates feed requirement.

Milk Composition

Water phase: Following constituents are dissolved in this aqueous phase

- Inorganic elements.
- Soluble nitrogenous substances – amino acids, creatine, urea.
- Water soluble protein – albumin.
- Lactose, enzymes.
- Water soluble vitamins – 'B' complex and detectable amounts of 'C'.
- In colloidal suspension of this phase are – inorganic substances mostly compounds of calcium, phosphorus and casein.
- Dispersed through aqueous phase is a suspension of minute milk fat globules.

Fat phase: Following constituents make up such phase

- Triglycerols make up 98 % of fat phase.

- The remainder being composed of certain fat associated substances – phospholipids, cholesterol, fat soluble vitamins, pigments, traces of protein and heavy metals.

The fat-phase is usually referred to simply as **"FAT"** and the remaining constituents other than water, are classed as **"Solids Not Fat" [SNF]**.

Sources of milk constituents

Various precursors are selectively absorbed from the blood and then these are utilized for the synthesis of major milk constituents in the udder. There are certain proteins, minerals and vitamins which are simply transferred directly from the blood to the milk by selective filtering action of udder.

- Milk proteins : Casein is the dominating protein in milk among others. The next protein in greatest amount is β-lactoglobulin.
- Lactose : This is the only carbohydrate in milk with the exception of glucose and few oligosaccharides.
- Milk fat : This consists of a mixture of tri-acylglycerols, which has predominant saturated (for example palmitic acid) and unsaturated (for example oleic acid, with small contributions from linoleic and linolenic acids).
- Minerals : Among major elements, milk contains calcium, phosphorus, sodium, magnesium, chloride and there are some twenty five trace elements in milk. Very small amounts of metalloids-boron, arsenic, silicon and halogens-fluorine, bromine and iodine are also included.

Considerable selectivity of udder

The inorganic constituents of milk are absorbed directly from blood by udder. The udder is capable of blocking the entry of some elements – selenium, fluorine, but allows the passage of zinc and molybdenum.

Transfer of substances between blood and milk is abnormal

The iron content of **Colostrum**, the milk produced in the immediate *postpartum* period, may be up to fifteen times that of normal milk.

- Vitamins are not synthesized in udder and therefore, they are absorbed from the blood. 'B' complex has the large range – thiamine, riboflavin, nicotinic acid, B_6, pantothenic acid, biotin, folacin, choline, B_{12} and inositol. Small amounts of vitamin C, D and traces of vitamin E, K occur in milk.

Milk has considerable vitamin A potency

This is due to the presence of vitamin A and carotene.

Milk yield drops on low feed intake

Restriction of feed intake has a profound influence upon both the yield and the composition of milk. It has been observed that milk yield drops to the tune of 0.5 kg per milking within three days upon fasting of cows. Simultaneously, solids-not-fat (SNF) and fat contents rise to about twice their previous levels. Obviously, the reduced yield results into concentration of milk. There is more influence on the SNF due to limitation of energy portion of diet.

Lactose concentration: The major determinant of the osmotic pressure of milk-lactose concentration showed little change. There might have been increased gluconeogenesis (formation of glucose from non-carbohydrate) from amino acids, owing to a reduced propionate (C_3) supply on low energy diets. That is why most of the fall in protein content. This might have reduction in the supply of amino acids to the udder and low protein synthesis.

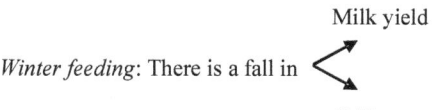

Winter feeding: There is a fall in Milk yield

SNF content, and this decline is prominent in the later period.

When the cows are allowed access to spring pasture, then

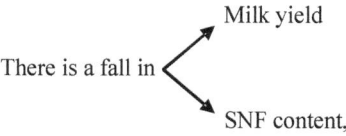

There is a fall in Milk yield

SNF content,

Experimentally, it was shown that such increases do not take place and indeed the opposite effect may be produced, where levels of winter feeding are high. Therefore, winter feeding of dairy cows appeared to be frequently inadequate.

Change of feeding in spring: This is frequently accompanied by a fall in the fat content of the milk.

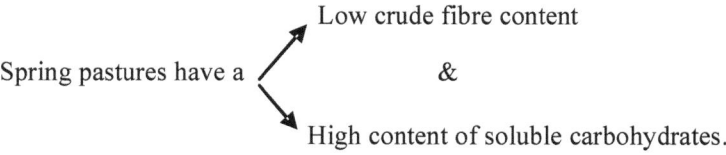

Spring pastures have a Low crude fibre content & High content of soluble carbohydrates.

Other diets having similar characteristics also bring about a decline in milk fat. These diets have a low ratio of roughage to concentrate and this could be due to very finely ground feed.

Lowered fat contents: These are usually accompanied by changes in the fatty acid composition with a

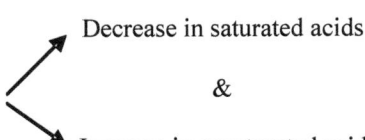

Decrease in saturated acids

&

Increase in unsaturated acids (particularly the 9 – Octadecenoic).

The changes in fat content and composition are associated with changes in rumen fermentation patterns. The buffering power of rumen – fluid is diminished because low fibre diets fail to stimulate salivary secretion. Pronounced peaks of acid production are exhibited with very low pH values, when such diets are often fermented rapidly. As a result, there is :

a) Inhibition of the activity of the cellulolytic fibre digesting microbes and that of -
b) Various starch utilizers encouraged.

The balance of volatile fatty acids in the rumen shows the reflection of above changes.

On the high fibre diets, the **molar proportions of volatile fatty acids** would be about :

i) 0.70 acetic acid (C_2)
ii) 0.18 propionic acid (C_3)
iii) 0.12 butyric acid (C_4)

[Together with a number of higher acids present in small amounts only].

The molar proportion of acetic acid falls and in extreme cases may be less than 0.4, when the fibre content of the diet is reduced and that of concentrates is enhanced. There would be decrease in butyric acid and increase in propionic acid with the above fall. The molar proportion would be 0.45 of the total acids present and the concentration of valeric acid may also increase side by side. Diets containing high proportions of carbohydrates (as with starch in flaked maize), the ratio of acetate to propionate as well as fat content may be effectively reduced.

The fat content of the diet is boosted

By feeding supplementary compound feeds: The dietary fat can be considered as a **source of energy.** It has been observed that milk yield drops, when the fat is replaced by an isocaloric amount of starch in the diet. High yielders require higher levels of dietary fat, but the constraints of intake make it difficult to provide sufficient energy.

Low fat syndrome: This may be due to diets 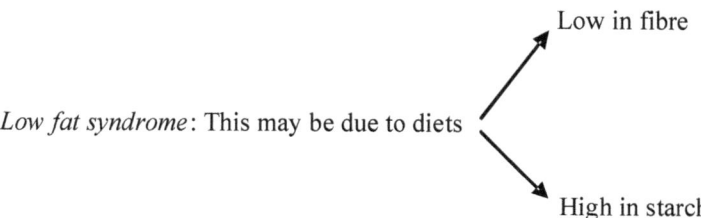 Low in fibre / High in starch

This situation may be corrected by increasing the fat content at the expense of starch fraction. Increased incorporation of long chain fatty acids of the dietary fat into milk fat helps in above correction. But *de novo* (within udder tissue) synthesis of short chain fatty acids and protein concentration (but not total protein secretion) go down. Unfortunately, by the addition of fat, fermentation and digestion of plant cell wall constituents in the rumen are impaired and hence, feed intake is depressed.

Unsaturated oils are less desirable

Feeding small quantity (200 g/d) of cod liver or herring oil can reduce fat content as much as 25 %. It is generally considered that for the daily ration of a lactating cow, less than 500 g of fat would suffice the purpose. For higher levels, **protected-fat** is advisable for the normal hydrogenation, solubilization and absorption to take place in the rumen. **Prills** (pellets) of calcium salts of fatty acids have turned out to be good for protection of fat. In addition the release of free fatty acids into rumen, are capable of **'fixation of calcium'** upon ingestion of fat. This prevents rumen microbes to utilize for their own good. This is not happening with **calcium soaps**. When prills are used, some energy – requirement may be met with dietary fat.

There is a profound influence on the composition of milk fat due to the nature of the dietary fat. The proportions of acids upto palmitic acid are increased in milk fat by the diets rich in these acids, at the expense of C_{18} acids. Increased yields of Oleic and Stearic acids with associated decreases in shorter chain acids (particularly palmitic) are resulted by the dietary fats rich in saturated and unsaturated acids. Because of **extensive hydrogenation** occurring in the rumen, the secretion of linoleic and linolenic acids is not affected. According to some indications, acetate : propionate ratio is affected in the rumen by polyunsaturated C_{18} acids. **Soybean oil** can markedly reduce the ratio of acetate to propionate. This oil is rich in linoleic acid. Activity in adipose tissue of enzymes involved in fatty acid and triacylglycerol synthesis is increased by those diets, which reduce milk fat. The activity of such enzymes occurs in udder tissue in a lesser degree at the same time. As a result, due to the use of acetate for fatty acid synthesis in the adipose tissue, the amount of acetate available for milk fat synthesis is reduced. A similar influence on the level of plasma free fatty acids would be there by the stimulation of triacyl glycerol synthesis. Low density lipoproteins are synthesized in the liver and their supply to udder for fat synthesis would thus be reduced. Finally, the precursors for milk fat synthesis would be used less efficiently due to reduced supply in the udder. The increased glucogenic nature of the acid mixture absorbed from the rumen on low-fat producing diets get support by the finding-intravenous infusions of glucose reduce plasma glyceride concentration.

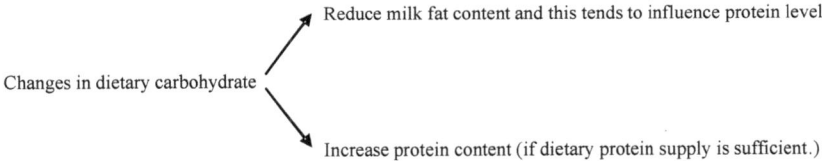

Such influence requires about three weeks making clear it. Certain glucogenic amino acids (such as glutamate) get sparing influence from propionic acid production on such diets. More of these glucogenic amino acids are then available to udder for protein synthesis. On such diets, the increased intake of energy would have the same effect.

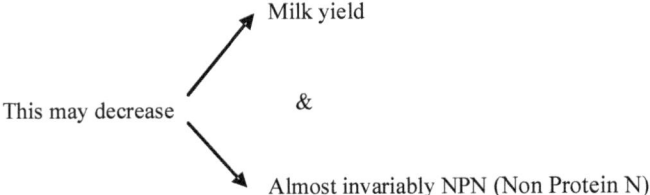

Reduction in dietary protein level

Protein intake upto 60 % of requirement, there is no issue for protein. This is perhaps due to an insufficiency of essential amino acids – methione > threonine > tryptophan.

Chapter 13

Examining Dairy Farm Management Closely

Ideas, materials, facilities, processes and labour are clubbed together to produce a worthwhile product-**milk** successfully and this may be the art and science of management. In other words, we put together the inputs-soil, labour, hay, fertility, silage into milk and such transformations are the result of a purposeful and premeditated action-management and not just by *happenstance*.

Decision making role of dairy farm manager

Manager of dairy farm decides :

- What to do !
- How to do !
- When to do !

For answering the above, the manager must plan to co-ordinate, organize, control and direct his supportive staff. For accomplishing his targets, the manager must gather information about all resources available, application of new technologies, different options of market outlets and sources of capital credit needed. He should be able to establish targets to be achieved. Obstacles or 'stumbling blocks' are always there which hinder progress towards goals. Therefore, these have to be identified. He should be able to compare alternative options of realizing targets, considering the each one in terms of income potential, the capital needed, the labour required. Then choosing the best plan of action and put that option into operation. The manager should be able to assume responsibility for the consequences of actions taken. Later, he should evaluate and measure results. His accomplishments may be assessed in the light of standards of performance. Not only that, but also to keep a vigil on production level, labour efficiency, cost, investments etc. He must keep the operating system flexible so that he may take advantage of new developments to be applicable in his plans.

For every decision made above

All the above operations may be undertaken routinely, should there be any problem, may be accordingly taken careof with some reasoning and planning. Some major decisions can also be taken :
- Buying a farm
- Closing a long – range plan of operation or,
- Making a major adjustment in operation.

Points to ponder about management

A farm manager should be well versed with many kinds of information affecting the milk production and for guiding management decisions, following are some of the tools :

a) **Farm records:** A system of accounting for a dairy farm is very important, so that milk production of any consequence can be operated successfully. Following are few important types of records -
   i) Complete inventories: This includes a summary of all assets, debts and net worth incurred at the beginning and end of each year.
   ii) Production records: This includes main animal products and their by-products.
   iii) Current expenditures and receipts: This includes quantities sold.
   iv) An annual production and financial summary
   v) An analysis of the year's record: This is to probe strong and weak points of production and to serve as a guide to wiser adjustments.

b) **Comparative budgeting :** For comparative alternative system of organizing overall farm production, this is the first and effective way, from the stand point of capital, requirements, labour as well as net income potential. Long-run expectations of yields and costs are the basis for such budgets.

c) **Annual budgeting :** In an operating system, this is a **"must"** to guide year to year adjustments. The latest outlook for yields and prices are the basis for annual budgets. They give future projections about production and allow one to correct mistakes in judgment before they happen. Or coming year's milk production is pre-viewed, which often allow one to **correct** mistakes in judgment **before** they happen.

d) **Partial budgeting :** For comparing the costs and returns from alternative adjustments in some part of farm production, this would be *shorter process*, such as the **"pros and cons"** of some new technology.

So, what is the conclusion!

- Reliable information must be the basis of major responsibility of farm manager as a planner.
- It is worthwhile repeating that all kinds of budgets used in planning for future should be :
  i) Careful analysis of our own records
  ii) A study of analysis from similar farming operations and
  iii) An up-to-date knowledge of the results of new research would provide the data needed.

Care of the cow and calf during and after parturition

Proper care and efficient management of the herd, is the key attribute for successful dairying. The dairy farm manager should pay special attention to cows in gestation period during and after calving, lest he would commit mistakes which would be very dear. Following may be some points to be gathered for guidance of care for cow and its calf.

Caring the cow

Following are some salient points for attention :

- **Gestation period :** If breeding records have been kept properly, the expected date can be calculated to within one to ten days. Generally, a dairy cow carries her calf on an average of 280 days.
- **Isolation of pregnant cows :** Advanced pregnant cows may be separated from rest of the herd and let them live in an isolated safety. This is just to prevent them from being injured by slipping on stable floors or by crowding through door ways or mounting cows or bulls that are in heat.
- **Symptoms that an animal is about to calve :** These include swelling of the udder, swelling of vulva and dropping away ligaments around the tail head. At that time, such pregnant cows should be housed in calving pen. That takes about a couple of hours for calving. The room should be neat and clean, well ventilated, well disinfected and bedded. Another way could be to have a small well grassed pasture, which should be free from trash or manure and close to frameshed (to get some observation), makes a good calving place during summers.
- **Some assistance always pays a helping-hand during parturition :** Generally, healthy vigorous domesticated animals don't require any assistance in the actual act of parturition. But, it is advisable that some

helping hand is always better, should some emergency arise. It has been observed that the front feet of calf appear first and thereafter the nose during parturition. If the labour prolongs for more than four hours, veterinary aid is called for.

- **After parturition :** The flanks, exterior of genitalia, tail should be washed with warm clean water containing some amount of potassium permanganate or *neem* leaves boiled in water. Such antiseptic wash adds to hygienic condition. The dam may be given warm jaggery-water to drink. Milking the cow partially is important to avoid **milk-fever** after parturition. The udder should not get any type of injury. The cow should be prevented from licking or ingestion of the placenta, because such practice adversely reduce milk yield due to excessive protein intake.

- **Feeding the dam :** In the beginning **bran-mash** moistened with lukewarm water provides **laxative effect**. Some green grass may also add to above due to fibre. After a couple of days', bran, oats, linseed mash may be replaced for bran mash. Healthy cows may not get affected during the first few days of nutrition at the time of calving. However, the amount of concentrates may be gradually increased to its normal requirement in the first fortnight.

- **Clinical aspects :** Following are some problems which may be needing veterinarian's attention :

  i) **Dystokia :** Abnormal presentation is probable, if the labour prolongs for more than four hours.

  ii) **Milk fever :** Controversy exists as to whether or not the udder should be milked out before calving. Hence, partial milking would be safe. The milker should not have old nails or ensure any such situation, which may injure the swollen udder.

  iii) **Mastitis :** There are always dangers that high productive cows will develop such problem and therefore, regular tests should be carried out by veterinarian.

  iv) **Expelling of placenta beyond twelve hours :**

  a) Within 2-4 hours: The placenta will normally leave the cow.

  b) Between 8-12 hours: If placenta is not expelled, then administer **Ergot** mixture.

  c) Beyond 12 hours: Apply manual help by a veterinarian. [When placenta (after birth) has been discharged, it should immediately be buried deeply. As has been mentioned above that dam should not lick or ingest placenta, because such practice adversely reduce milk yield due to excessive protein intake].

Simplifying management of new born calf

Following are some points which may be taken care – of :

- **All mucous to be removed :** The care – taker should make sure that all mucous is removed from the nose and mouth, immediately after the calf is born. So that, calf breathes normally. Otherwise, alternately compressing and relaxing the chest walls with the hands should be done for artificial respiration after calf is layed on its side.

- **Naval care :** At the time of birth, 'tincture of iodine' is applied at naval, dusted with boric acid powder. The long cord is swiped off about two inches from the body before above application. The naval cord is neither allowed to drain nor tied.

- **Let calf stand on its own :** The new born calf, under most conditions, would be on its feet and ready for suckling within an hour. Some helping hand is good at this juncture. The attendant should clean the udder before calf-nursing, so that much of the infection could be prevented before hand.

- **About colostrum :** Following are couple of points which are very crucial for calf feeding :

    a) The dairy farm manager should ensure that the calf gets first milk colostrum at least for 48 hours. The calf is protected against diseases by the gamma-globulins (antibodies) of colostrum. It also shows laxative effect which is good for the calf.

    It is believed that the colostrum is such mother-nature's formula, which has not yet been duplicated. And whatever diseases the dam might have encountered during her life till parturition, would not happen with the calf, due to presence of antibodies for all those diseases.

    b) About ten per cent of the calf's weight per day, milk is being fed and gradually increased upto a maximum of five litres per day.

    c) More information is available elsewhere in this chapter [page 73].

- **Weaning:** There is variation in such practice regarding the best time to remove the calf from dam:

    a) Generally the calf is separated from its mother after the first feeding, because **it simplifies the management and reduces the feed and labour costs for rearing.**

    b) Some dairy men allow the calf to remain with its dam for a couple of days in the beginning or until the milk is suitable to put in the regular supply. That won't make much difference as to when the calf is removed from its dam.

- **Separate pen or stall for calf:** Such practice allows better attention to individual calves. After about eight weeks of age, they may be mingled up in a group. Some other measures may be taken as :
  a) Identifying the calf by **tattooing**.
  b) Periodically **body weight is recorded.**
  c) **Dehorning** may be carried out within ten days. Because, **the horn-buttons are not attached with the skull by then.**
  d) **Extra teats** beyond the normal four are unsightly and hence should be removed. Because, such extra teats create difficulty at the time of milking

- **Clinical aspects :** Following are some situations, where a veterinarian's attention may be sought :
  a) **Scouring :** This happens when milk allowance is high and hence, this may be reduced to half litre or less until the calf recovers.
  b) **Haemorrhagic Septicemia (H.S.) :** This is practiced at the age of fifteen days, when about 35 ml of H.S. serum is inoculated into the calf for bacterial disease.
  c) **Anthrax** and **Black quarters (B.Q.) :** At the age three months, the calf is vaccinated for Anthrax spore vaccine (living) and thereafter, they are vaccinated for B.Q.

Good animals are raised, not purchased

Raising the dairy calf

Future of any dairy farm herd depends on how calves are raised. However good may be a scientific breeding system, the outcome – a calf should be properly fed and managed, so that it may attain to its full potential. Irrespective of high pedigree, the dairyman has to raise one's own calves to make a good herd.

System of calf rearing

There are mainly the following two kinds of calf rearing :
  a) The dam and calf are together a little before and after milking.
  b) The calf is taken away from its dam after a couple of days' of parturition. That means, calf is allowed to be with its mother till the colostrum-period. After this, it would be the sole responsibility of dairyman for feeding and

management of the calf and this is called the **'Weaning system'**. Because of multifarious advantage, this system is getting more popular in :
i) Military dairy farms
ii) Government and progressive farms.

On the scientific lines, calves are raised as following :

i) **Calf before birth :** Care is taken for a dairy calf, even before it is born. Therefore, pregnant cows are fed properly, so that well-nourished calves are born. Special care must be taken to feed the cows liberally during the four months before calving. This nourishes the growing tissues of the calf as well as the dam to withstand the strain of parturition normally. Such cows should have free access to grazing fields. Still a couple of kgs of grain mixture in addition to green legumes, would add to her proper health.

ii) **Calf after birth :** Following couple of measures are important :
   a) Treatment of calf : After parturition, the calf should be able to breathe comfortably. For this purpose, the slimy mucous is cleaned with a clean and soft towel or smooth dry paddy straw, just as imitation of the way the cow licks, because dryness is important.
   b) Naval cord : Cut half inch from the body and apply incture of iodine (30 %).

iii) **Feeding the calves :** Here, emphasis is given on colostrum feeding –
   a) Colostrum feeding: Following its birth, calf must receive two litres of colostrum daily for three days [its digestibility increases at about 38^0 C (100^0F)]. Any excess colostrum may be fed to other calves in the herd, in amount of whole milk normally fed. Still if some of the colostrum is left, it should be freezed for later feeding. The idea is that, none of the colostrum should be wasted.
   b) Importance of colostrum : Following are some advantages of colostrum

i) There is higher proportion of gamma-globulin in the colostrum than normal milk has. This proportion is the source of antibodies, which protect the calf from many infections.

Level of g-globulin	Stage
0.97 mg / ml	At birth
16.55 mg / ml	At 12 hrs., Ist feeding.
28.18 mg / ml	On 2nd day (peaks) [This level continues till 'Reticulo endothelial system' of the calf start functioning to produce antibodies]

ii) The protein content of colostrum is five times of normal milk. It is also rich in iron, copper, manganese, magnesium.
iii) It contains ten times the amount of vitamin A found in normal milk.
iv) It is also rich in riboflavin, choline, thiamine, and pantothenic acid.
v) It helps the digestive tract to clear off the faecal material due to its property of laxative action.

Teaching the calf to drink milk

If the calf is with the mother, then it is a natural instinct, which automatically leads the calf to reach the udder within a short period or may have little assistance. But, in weaning system, considerable **patience** is required in teaching the calf to have milk from the **pail.**

One may pour some of the mother cow's milk into clean pail by allowing the calf to suck the finger of the feeder, so that its head may be guided into the pail and then hand of the feeder can be gradually lowered into the bucket and submerged in the milk sufficiently deep to allow a little milk to be taken by the calf. By continuous feeding, it will learn to drink.

In some farms, they prefer to use **nipple pail** for feeding the calf during first four weeks of its life. Such pail is equipped with a rubber nipple, from which the calf sucks. It has the advantage in that, the calf takes the milk more slowly, and **is therefore**, less likely to have digestive upsets. These nipple pails should be cleaned, washed thoroughly after each feeding.

Feeding whole milk

Following points may be remembered :
a) Milk from the calf's mother may be provided, as far as possible.
b) Immediately after it is drawing, it should be fed.
c) On other situations, the milk may be provided at body temperature.
d) Frequency of milk feeding may be four at equal intervals upto the age of seven days and then twice daily.

Feeding skim milk

Large quantities of fat-less milk after centrifugal separation are available on many farms, which can be fed to calves and other livestock. After two weeks of their age, excellent dairy calves can be raised on such skim milk as per the feeding schedule. Such milk has less than one per cent fat and almost no soluble vitamins.

Feeding dried skim milk, whey or butter milk

Depending on availability at a reasonable rate of above products, they can be mixed with water and after warming at 100°F (about 38°C), may be fed to calves.

Feeding calf starters

Following measures may be adopted :

- Mainly dairy farmers turned their calves to 'calf-starter' method owing to the expenses and labour involved.
- A mixture consisting of ground farm grains, protein feeds, vitamins, minerals and antibiotics constitute calf-starter.
- After a calf attains the age of two weeks, some amount of whole milk may be replaced with calf-starter.
- For promoting better growth and vigour, milk feeding is especially helpful. Another reason of milk-feeding is that, some calves *do not eat freely on 'starter'*. It may have to be continued for a long time.
- After each milk-feeding, one may rub a small amount of **'starter'** on the calf's mouth, for some days, so that the calf would be accustomed to it.
- After reaching four months of age, one may **discontinue** above practice and shift the calves to a **'growing'** grain ration.

Feeding grain mixture

Some of the following observations may be given consideration :

- It has been observed that consumption of both **grain and milk** results in the better growth and **greater resistance** to calf – **ailments.**
- At the age of ten days, feeding of grain mixture may be started.
- For getting the calves **familiar** to grain mixture, place a small handful of grain mixture in the **used pail.**
- Some amount of grain – mixture may be offered to calf, immediately after feeding milk.
- Average **thumb rule** for grain mixture requirement:

Oats	=	35 %	Barley	=	10 %
Linseed cake	=	5 %	Groundnut cake	=	20 %
Wheat bran	=	30 %.			

Another way of feeding mixture may be as following :

Groundnut cake = two parts
Wheat bran = two parts
Linseed meal = one part

Feeding silage

These are some of the measures of feeding :

- Small amounts of silage may be given to calves, at their 3-6 months of age.
- Feed 1 kg/d to calves of 3 months and then gradually the amount is increased by 500 g/d for each month of calfage.
- Quality silage be ensured (avoiding mouldy/damaged silage leads to indigestion).

Feeding after discontinuing milk

Good leguminous hay, concentrates, good pasture are among the best feeds, which may be fed liberally, after the milking is discontinued (that is, calves should not be neglected after milk is being discontinued).

Pasturing calves

This area also needs attention in the following ways:

a) Calves should be accessible to independent pasture, from those of older animals. This is just to avoid –
   - Any **physical injury** by the older animals,
   - To prevent the calves from **exciting** the cows by **running** about among them.

b) In addition to pasture, the calves may be allowed to a :

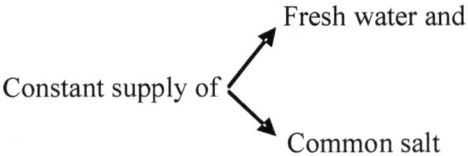

c) Some **steamed bone meal** of good quality as mineral supplement may also be given to calves. This is important for such pasture consisting of non – legume grass growing on an acid soil.

Providing minerals

Following points may be thought for :

- During milk feeding, there is **no problem** for calcium or phosphorus deficiency.
- High quality legumes are excellent sources of calcium, and grain mixtures are good for phosphorus.
- If good feed is poorly available then, at rate of 2 % mineral mixture (of bureau of Indian standards grade) may be given.
- In addition, iodized salt is also essential.

Supplying antibiotics

For example :

Aureomycin they increase growth rate of dairy heifers without any apparent effect upon :

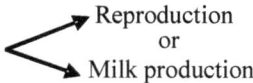

They may be fed in consultation with veterinarian. Advantages of such feeding are :

- Appetite increases
- Number of Calf – scour cases would go down.
- They have smoother hair coats.

Housing the calf

Some planning may be as following :

- This is for shelter against inclemency's of weather – Sun, rain, storm etcetera.
- Open exercise paddock continuing to their housing is desirable.
- Calf pens should be located close to cow sheds and clean drinking water be always accessible.
- Separate housing may be planned as under :
  a) Under 3 months
  b) 3-6 months
  c) Over 6 months till weaning.

Dehorning the calf

Removal of horn-roots from dairy animals by treating with a chemical, mechanical or electrical devices, is called as dehorning. Such practice is very painful in yearlings or older animals and may result in considerable bleeding. Dehorning is therefore, practiced in ten days old calves, because **the horn buttons do not become attached to the skull.**

Advantages of dehorning

- Dehorned animals are safe to handle by the operators.
- Such animals do not inflict injury to each other, hence economic losses are avoided
- They require less room in the sheds.
- There is no need of defending themselves. Afterall, they would be in harmony with each other and moreover they are under the supervision of care – takers.
- Their productive performance **would speak for itself**, rather than any show – off in any exhibition or cattle shows.

Castrating the bull calf (♂): or male

This is the un-sexing of not only male but also female animal by way of removal of both testicles or ovaries respectively. Such surgical operations are very common as well as old. This method is just to prevent reproduction, so that there may be faster gains and animals become docile and easier to handle. In western or gulf countries, such male animals are raised for more desirable type of meat production. Calves, lambs, swine may be castrated at about 10 wks, 2 wks, 1 wk respectively.

Scientific method of castrating

Since the recent past, they have been using a strong and tight rubber ring around the cord at an early age of the calf; thereby a constant pressure is being created in males. When the testicles have been absorbed, **the ring drops down**.

Handling cross-bred cows

India is using some exotic breeds of cattle for example – Jersey, Holstein Fresian, Red dane, Brown swiss etc. for cross – breeding purpose. These breeds have following performance :

- Holstein happens to be the highest milk yielder (> 6000 litres / lactation), with low fat (3.5 %).
- Jersey is small sized with a little low milk yield (about 4000 litres / lactation), with a little high fat content (4.5 %).
- Other two above breeds fall in between these two regarding their milk production and fat content.

Right now, it is suggested that

To Maintain :

- 50 % exotic blood in the cross-bred animals in **plains** of India, whereas
- 62.5 % in the **hilly** areas.

Such level may be achieved by using **inter-mating** or **forward crossing of** F_2 generations respectively.

Following suggestions may be observed

i) **Summer stress:** During summer months of April to August, the milk yield of cross bred cows is likely to be affected. At extremely high temperature, there may be :

- Degeneration of testicular epithelium in the male animals, which may lead to inferior quality of semen production.
- Feed intake is reduced in such cross bred animals due to high environmental temperature. This situation may be partly avoided by providing ample shady trees during summer months.

ii) **Disease control:** Cross breds have less-disease resisting ability with respect to Indian breed animals. Because of following reasons :

- Cross breds are prone to **Foot and mouth disease,** hence such stocks may be **vaccinated** for all contagious fatal diseases.
- Mastitis is also frequently observed in such cross breds and therefore, it becomes imperative for the owners to get their cross breds checked periodically.
- They are sensitive to Parasitic infections too. Obviously, right from the early age, rigorous preventive measures may be attended.

Feeding Piperazine compounds would be helpful once during

i) For young animals:

   1-2 months, followed by

   3-4 months

   5-6 months

ii) For adults: Intervention of Veterinarian is called for, because high mortality is observed in cross breds due to parasitic infections (as compared to Indian pure breeds).

iii) **Nutritional aspect:** Following strategy may be taken care of :
   - Nutritonal requirements have to be higher for such high yielders.
   - Only succulent fodders are not sufficient to cater their energy needs.

Hence, supplementation of 'higher energetic concentrate mixtures' becomes imperative. As a **"Thumb – rule"**, one tenth of its body weight, green fodders as well as 'energy – rich' concentrates may be fed to above animals, for the sake of economy.

For bullocks: They may be utilized for hard ploughing work during the early morning and evening timings of summer months. During cooler months of the year, that would be just normal practice.

Housing for dairy cattle

Proper planning and adequate space for dairy cattle is important for an efficient management of cattle. This would result in saving of labour charges and thus, improve profit of the owner. For proper provision of comfortable accommodation of dairy cattle, care should be ensured during construction of houses, with regard to :

- Proper sanitation
- Durability
- Production of clean milk under convenient and economic conditions.

Location of dairy building

Following dots may be considered :

a) **Local geography and channel for carrying off liquid:** Dairy building should be at higher elevation than the surrounding areas to offer a good slope for rainfall and drainage for the dairy wastes to avoid stagnation within the buildings.

b) **Foundation land:** In order to avoid the soil to be susceptible for considerable swelling during rainy season as well as with numerous cracks and fissure, the land may be prevented to get dehydrated or desiccated.

c) **Long axis of dairy be set in North-South direction :** This is just to have maximum benefit of the Sun in the North and minimum in the South. Protection from prevailing strong wind currents whether hot or cold. However, the placement of the building would facilitate the direct Sun light to reach the platforms, gutters and feeding-mangers in the cattle shed.

d) **Electricity and water supply :** These days the modern dairy always handles electric equipments, which are also economical, therefore, it is desirable to have an adequate supply of electricity. Abundant supply of fresh, clean and soft water should be available at cheaper rate.

e) **Marketing :** Dairy owner may be able to bring his products regularly and sell at a reasonable price.

f) **Relative position of Centre cross-alley of cow barn :** This may be located at hand to feed storages, hay stacks, silo, near to milking parlour, the stall area, the manure pits for the optimum utilization of labour. Sufficient space per cow and well arranged feeding-mangers and resting areas would lead to greater production, convenience of workforce, reducing feed expenses.

Comfortable housing facilities ease out the animals to move in or out of standing space or mangers, open paddock for water etc. However, a little close confinement or restrictions at milking time. There are two types of dairy housing systems :

i) Loose housing system (economical)
ii) Conventional dairy barn (expensive)

Loose housing dairy barn

This is a type of barn where animals are having restrictions during milking and at the time of treatment. Otherwise, they are let loose all the time. This system appears to be very economical. Following are some important aspects of these raising dairy cattle :

a) The animals are **at liberty** and at their own free will even with minimum grazing. Hence, such barn proves to be profitable.

b) For better health and production, the animals get ample **physical exercise**.

c) **Cost** of construction significantly lower.

d) It is flexible with any **future expansion** without many changes even on the existing infrastructure.

e) **Rendering** of overall management is better.

Other provisions

There is availability of milking barns, calf pens, calving pens, store rooms etc. in such kind of system. Each shed would be having arrangement for feeding manger, drinking area, loitering area too. Following construction, technical matters may be kept in mind :

Shed : This may be cemented or brick paved and therefore, easily cleaned.

Floor : This would be rough for avoiding slipping of animals.

Drain : This would be shallow preferably covered with removable tiles.

Roof : Corrugated cement sheets of asbestos or brick rafters may be used for gable shaped roofs. This would be little expensive.

Walls : Animals would automatically lie down to have the protection from the walls.

[All the above constructive materials, different dimensions of buildings would be dependent on the market prevailing value, size of the herd as well as choice of the owners].

Conventional dairy barn

This kind of barn facilitates the cattle more protection from adverse climatic conditions, the system is a little expensive though. Different sheds are constructed for cattle based on different purposes as following :

Cow sheds : These are arranged in single or double row depending on the number of cows, less than ten or more respectively. Generally, not more than eighty cows are housed in one building and they may be arranged to face as per the choice of the owner :

i) Tail to tail or
ii) Head to head

Time motion studies in dairies

It has been observed that :

15 % of the expended time is spent **in front of the cow**.

60 % of the time is spent **behind the cows**. This duration is four times more than the time spent in front of them.

25 % of the time is spent in **other parts** of the barn and milk house.

Tail to tail arrangement

- The wide middle alley facilitates in cleaning and milking the cows.
- The head care – taker can inspect a greater number of milkmen while milking.
- It would be easier to monitor the animals for any kind of minor disease or any change in the hind quarters.

Face to face arrangement

- Feeding can be carried out without back tracking and hence, easier to do so.
- For narrow barn, such arrangement is helpful. Also, cows feel easier to get into their stalls.
- The gutter gets plenty of air, Sun – shine from outside.

Stall design

It is the choice of dairy owner whether he prefers stanchion or tie stall. Whatever may be the designs, the idea is to protect the cows of their udder and teats from being stepped on by other cows. The cows may be allowed to the greatest possible freedom and with much of the comfort. Also, it is important to line them up, such that most of the droppings and urine go to the gutter.

Other sheltering

Calving boxes, isolation boxes, sheds for young stocks may have good provisions for nursing for milk, manger for feed, alleys, manure-gutter, doors in the proper order, proper ventilation, paddock etc.

Calvin boxes

These would be separate from milking cow shed, otherwise may cause instant milk secretion and there may be spread of disease, like **contagious abortion** in the heard. Hence, special accommodation in the form of loose boxes enclosed from all sides with door be provided to all parturient cows along with sufficient ventilation for air and light.

Isolation boxes

Animals suffering from infectious diseases must be segregated soon from the rest of the herd (in quarantine), away from other barns, should be self – contained and should have separate connection to drainage disposal system.

Bull – bullock shed

The accommodation may have provision for :
- Safety and ease in handling.
- Comfortable shed for protection from adverse weather conditions.
- Free access to exercise yard.

A bull should not be kept in confinement particularly on hard floors. Because such a confinement without adequate exercise leads to overgrowth of the hooves, creating difficulty in mounting and loss in the breeding power of the bull. Adequate arrangement for ventilation for light and air. Shed should have manger, water trough. If possible, **water and feed be served without actually entering the bull house.** Free access to an exercise yard provided with a strong fence or a boundary, high enough, such that bull may not jump over. The bull should be able to observe other animals from a distance, so that it may not feel isolated. The exercise yard should have **service crate** via a swing gate, which saves the use of an attendant to bring the bull to service crate.

The identity of an animal

For a small herd, some dairymen name their cows which may serve purpose to some extent. But for pure breed animals and large herd, it is always necessary to mark each and every animal. The customary of marking is by :
- Tattooing, ear – tagging (for example notches),
- Neck, horn chains,
- Branding numbers on hips,
- Photos, colour sketches.

Ear – tagging
Number or letters are engraved on metal or plastic pieces, which are either self – piercing or they may require a hole in the ear, which is made with an ear – punch. Such tags are placed on the upper edge of the ear with the number on top and within **One third** of the way out from the base of the ear.

Tattooing
Here, light coloured ears are punctured with a die to make small holes, in the form of numbers or letters, through the skin. Thereafter, the holes are filled with tattoo ink. **Disadvantage** is that the animals have to be caught and for reading the marks, inside of the ear is cleaned.

Examining Dairy Farm Management Closely

Number tags

The neck chains have large metal or plastic tags to be read from a distance. The objectionable point is that, there may be a chance that they may be lost.

Branding

This is done preferably before the calf is weaned. A heated stamp or branding liquid may be used on the body, which causes partial burning of the tissue, producing a permanent scar at the lower part of thigh.

Ear – notching

The method is common in **swine** and **sheep**. Notches are put into the right or left ear to represent a number. Some dairymen would not be willing to **disfigure** the ears of their cattle in this way.

In poultry and sheep

Light **aluminum tags** are used as wing tags in poultry or as leg – band. In case of sheep, identification mark is used by means of **marking fluid**.

Record keeping

For proper monitoring of cow – herd, a fairly good record of following is important for a dairyman :

- The amount of feed given to cows in the herd,
- The amount of milk and butter fat produced in the farm.

Preserving records

Permanent records may be in the form of books, for example pedigree, breeding, property registration matters etc. Such methodology has the advantage of being safer. However, there are certain other routine or periodical recordings, which may be handled frequently and are in use at a particular need, they may be in loose books or files.

Cattle feed record (nutritional aspect)

It is important to maintain the records of production as well as feed consumed of a cow for the purpose of assessing profit she is making. In the large herds, it is also important to pen down the amount of feed that may be given to each cow should receive. But that is not possible to remember the amount of feed that me be given to each individual cow. For every fortnight, such kind of records is changed. Therefore, as per the production of individual cow, the recording may be **clipped near the feed bin**. The amount of **grain** may be weighed carefully at each feeding as per the clipped – sheet. However, roughages need not be weighed at each feeding, but once a month that may be weighed to have some idea, as to how much amount the cow might have consumed. Numbering different grain mixtures is routinely carried out in the large farms. The situation is different for calves, because they are fed skim milk, whole milk, hay or grain.

Breeding record

There are two ways to put up 'Service records' :

- **Bull wise:** Recording for **'a particular bull'** mating all cows are noted down.
- **Cow wise:** Recording for **'a particular cow'** being serviced by all bulls are jotted down.

Then again, **cross – checking** the combination of above both clarifies the exact position.

Handling the bull

Ringing

Ring in the nose of a bull is a safeguard to handle. They say each and every bull should have ring including a gentle bull. At 8 months of age, a copper ring is put in the nose of a bull. At 2 years of age, a larger gun – metal ring may be replaced under the supervision of a veterinarian.

Disadvantage: Due to some sudden jerk on the tight rope or getting the ring caught on something accidently, could be serious to cartilage. For example may cause tearing of the **septum** of his nose. Such method may not be always successful, because such single or double rings may give the animal considerable trouble in eating and may get caught on objects.

Trimming the feet

Longer hoofs are not only unsightly but may become so painful that the bull can not stand or walk squarely. This may lead to sore feet. After tying the animal in standing position, the hoofs may be trimmed with hoof – knife.

Trimming and polishing the horns

Horns can also be taken care with fine sand paper. Smooth off the dead tissue, but not across. After polishing, application of linseed oil and pumice stone is suggested.

Never trust a bull

Any bull should be handled in a firm manner because, many accidents had resulted from trusting the so-called **gentle bull**. Sometimes, *as a result of taking chances*, a person is very badly injured or killed. Even in the face of a docile life history, the bulls have an unpredictable viciousness of disposition probably unequalled by any of our domestic animals. Therefore, they may be easily labeled as the most dangerous beast on the farm. Additionally, when aroused, bulls should not be discounted due to their enormous strength and killing instinct. Therefore, they should be under absolute control, while taking them in public.

Bull should not put on fat

The bull should be allowed to move about and have regular exercise such that they may be vigorous at service. They should come from parents with a typical breed of high index of potential. Obviously, they should be free from communicable diseases.

[These days majority of farmers are going for artificial insemination of their cows.]

Teeth: Weapons of defense

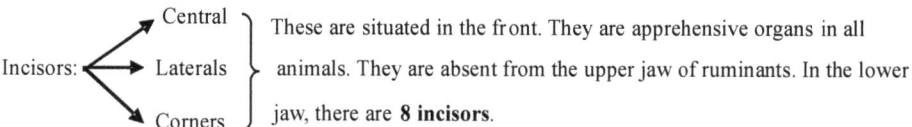

Incisors: Central, Laterals, Corners — These are situated in the front. They are apprehensive organs in all animals. They are absent from the upper jaw of ruminants. In the lower jaw, there are **8 incisors**.

For prehension, mastication, teeth are used by animals. **"Cheek teeth"** are:

In non – ruminants

Canines are behind the incisors and typical of carnivorous and omnivorous animals and mainly for fighting purpose.

In ruminants

Upper jaw: This has no canines, and in the :

Lower jaw: The canines have moved forward, assuming the function and shape of the incisors.

In all the domestic animals, there are two sets of teeth as following –

Ist Set: Consists of fewer teeth and appears early in life and is called – deciduous or temporary or milk teeth.

IInd Set: The first set is gradually replaced by the permanent dentition during the course of growth.

The deciduous dentition provides the young mammal with a fully functional, though smaller set of teeth that can be accommodated by its small jaws. As the jaws grow longer, new permanent teeth are added and the deciduous teeth are gradually replaced by permanent teeth. The eruption and wearing out of the incisors of the cattle are related to their age and its due to this fact that within certain limits, it is possible to estimate the age of domesticated animals.

Teeth of the cattle

In all ruminants, **"dental pad"** takes up the place of incisors in the upper jaw and in the lower jaw, the incisors are slightly movable in a direction. The 8 incisors are chisel shaped and do not have flat tables and infundibulum.

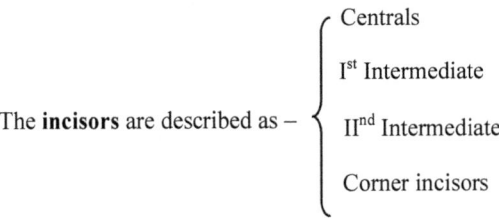

The canines are absent in all ruminants. The pre – molars and molars are somewhat chisel – shaped and progressively increase in size from Ist to last. The pre – molars and molars have well – formed **grinding surface**.

Age determination in cattle

By examining the teeth, the age estimation of our dairy cattle can be checked out.

About tooth	About approximate age
2 Central incisors	The calf is born with.
Other incisors start coming out	As the calf advances in age
Eruption of all the 8 temporary incisors are completed.	When the calf is 5 – 6 months old.
The above incisors are replaced by permanent teeth (these are smaller but broader with distinct neck between the root and crown. And appearance is off – white.	In due course of time, with the advancement.
Gradually, above teeth start wearing off	With the further advancement of age.
At 10 months	2 temporary incisors show signs of wearing.
At 15 months	2 lateral incisors start wearing off
At 1½ years	The whole set of milk teeth are flattened by the action of time.
At 2 years	The 2 central temporary incisors are replaced by the permanent ones.
At 3 years	The 2 intermediate incisors also get replaced.
At 4 years	The corner incisors are also replaced.
At 6 years	The entire set of 8 teeth is completely replaced by permanent teeth.
After 6 years, changes occur in the level of these permanent incisors.	
At 6 – 7 years	The central incisors get worn out.
At 7 – 8 years	The I^{st} intermediate incisor gets worn out.
At 8 – 10 years	The IInd intermediate incisor gets worn out.
By 11th year	The corner incisors get worn out
At the age of 11 years	Incisors become smaller due to wear and tear.
After 12 years	Incisor teeth become smaller due to wear and tear.
By the 12th year of age	The dental tables become square, instead of oval and the teeth stand apart leaving space between them.
After 12 years	Practically, age estimation by examining the teeth becomes difficult as well as the productive life of our dairy cattle also become lost.

Taking care of vices

There are certain bad habbits among the cattle, which create nuisance and therefore, they should be dealt from the first observation. Following are some such vices :

1. **Licking:** Calves, for example, during the milk – feeding period, start licking other calves. This results in the digestion of hair, which get trapped with the curdled milk in the stomach and forms hair balls. These balls continue to grow in size upon accumulation of more hair and lead to serious transmittable disorders.

Precautions
- After each feeding, a pinch of salt or mineral mixture may be rubbed on the tongue. On few applications, they will forget this habbit.
- Rope-net or wire-gauge muzzles may also be used.
- Young calves may be kept in the individual pens or tied at a distance.

2. **Suckling:** Cows suck themselves or other cows, heavy economic losses occur including contamination of udder or at times, indigestion of stomach. Why they do so !!! There is no satisfactory answer so far Psycological or Wat !!!

Precaution
- They may be kept in separate pens for preventing this perversion.
- A cradle or a bull ring may be put in the cow's nose and then 2-3 other rings are attached to it.
- A special ring that has some sharp progs soldered on to it. This method is also effective and does not interfere with the animal's normal eating.

3. **Kicking:** During milking, some cows kick the milker. This may be by nature vicious.

Precaution
- The cow's head may be tied high.
- Alternatively, a rope may also be tied around the body of the cow, just in front of the udder.
- Anti – linking chains can be used. A clamp fits over each hock and a chain fastens them together.
- A piece of rope is used to tie the hocks by making a loop like the '8', crossed between the two hocks to avoid slipping down the strap while struggling.

4. **Fence breaking:** They jump over the fences, may be due to the feeling that on the other side of the fence, the grass is greener or plenty.

Precaution: For such rough cows, proper hitching arrangements and good fences would be proper action.

Chapter 14

Feed Technology

When we talk about importance of feed technology in relation to animal productivity, feed represents the major cost in animal production as follows -

Domestic species	Feed representing on an average [% of the total production cost]
For sheep (typically consumes more **forage** than others)	55 % or more
For poultry	75 %
For Swine (pork)	70 %
For finishing cattle	60 %
For lactating cattle	70 %

Feed processing includes all operations necessary to achieve the maximum potential of nutritional value of a feed stuff. The process involves changing ingredients in such a manner as to maximize their natural value and the net returns from their use. Feed processing may be accomplished by Physical, Chemical, Thermal, Bacterial or other changes of a feed ingredient before it is fed. The primary reasons for processing feeds are to make changes in the moisture content, density of feed, particle size, palatability; or to make more profit, to improve nutrient availability, keeping quality; or to reduce storage - transportation space, cost, moulds, salmonella and other harmful substances. Detoxification of undesirable components because some feeds may contain toxic substances, the excess consumption of which may cause decreased nutritive value of the feeds or may injure some vital organs or even cause death. Some natural inhibitors in feedstuffs are as following :

Feed stuff	Inhibitor (s) or toxins	De-activating process
Cotton seed meal (binaula)	Gossypol (cycloprene fatty acid)	By adding iron salts for rupturing pigment glands.
Soybean meal (oil seed)	Saponin (pectin methyl esterase)	Limit amount Feed
Groundnut meal	Afflatoxin	Treat with NH_3 or NH_4OH
Raw fish	Thiaminase (enzyme)	Heating
Egg – albumin	Avidin (its one molecule binds three molecules of **Biotin**).	Heating.

Feed mill equipments

The milling industry has been concerned with "Grinding" – a process of particle size reduction. During earlier times, the same equipment was used

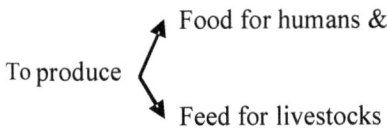

because, the process was basically 'grinding' of whole grains. As milling developed into the 'Modern Flour Industry', the milling process was extended to include :

Sieving	Heat conditioning
Purification to remo ve the bran and germ fractions to produce modern white – flour.	Recently, mill owners had started to add enriching ingredients.
Mixing	Pelleting
Flaking	Crumbling

Hammer mills

These are used for the grinding of both – grains and forages. The hammer mill consist of a cylinder – rotar made up of several plates, which are keyed to the main shaft or axle. Pins through these plates near the edge, carry the hammers, which are attached to them. Outside the rotating cylinder is a perforated steel screen. The holes in this screen may be as small as $1/32^{nd}$ inch or as large as two or more inches. Hammer mills may be of single, double or triple reduction type with either rigid or swinging hammers. The double or triple reduction types have knives or blunt disks on one side of the rotar to chop the longer stemmed materials, such as – corn fodder or alfa alfa (Lucerne) in contact with the hammers.

This type of mill is usually fed from a central opening, so the material being reduced, will come into contact with knives and disks first. It is assumed that most of the grinding occurs as the hammers strike the material in the air, as it falls into the mill. The hammer tip may travel at speeds of about 7000-25000 feet / minute. If the first impact of the hammers against the grain is missed, it rebounds and is again struck by the hammer tips. This process continues until all particles are reduced to a size that will allow them to pass through the screen (Fig. 3). A fan or blower is generally used for product transport after grinding. The fan may be connected to the same shaft that drives the hammer mill or it may be driven separately. In either situation, the fan requires about 25 – 30 % of horse power of the mill. The fan helps in product removal from the mill and also cools the stock being reduced.

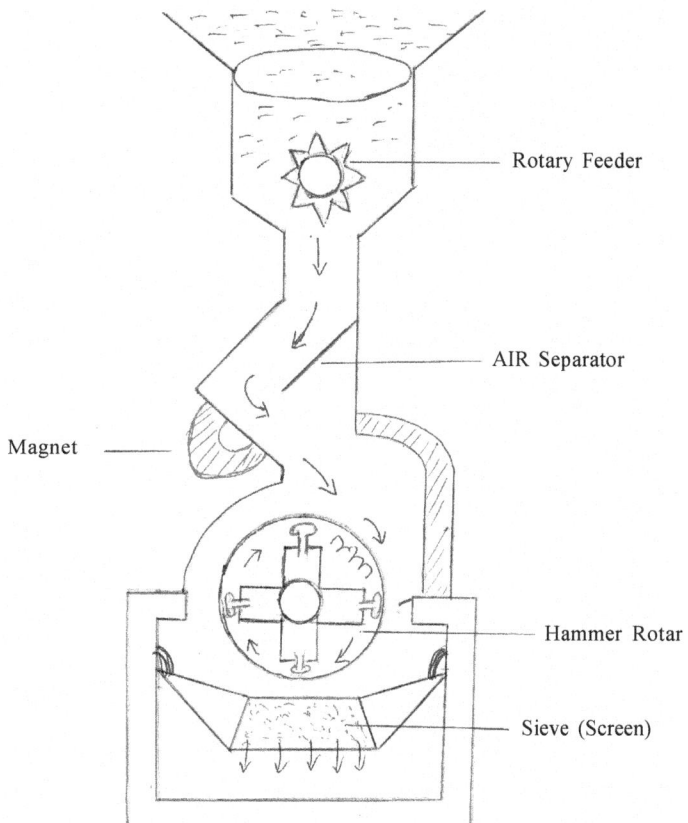

Fig. 3 : Vertical Mixer [Diagrammatic Representation]

Attrition mill

These are also called "Plate mills", consist of

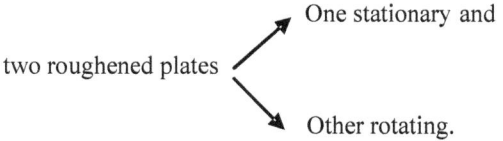

The material is fed between the plates and is reduced by cutting, crushing and shearing. The attrition mill is a heavy – duty commercial preparation of feed and food products. Each plate rotates and is driven independently with high speeds. In general, it can be said that :

Attrition is more efficient, when producing a **coarser** product &

Hammer mill is more efficient, when producing a **finer** product.

Attrition also produces a more uniform grind than hammer mill.

Roller mills

These are used in feed processing for crimping or crushing of grains :

a) The double roller mill is used for this purpose, which consists of two rolls rotating in opposite directions at the same speed. The material is crushed between rolls. Rolls are usually corrugated or serrated.

b) The roller mills used in the flour milling industry, have a slow roll and fast roll. They may or may not be corrugated. Such rolls have **"speed differential"**, therefore cutting and shearing will take place. If the rolls are operated at the same speed, the reduction is mostly by crushing. Roller mills may have one or two pairs of rolls in strand or set.

Steaming

Steaming may be used along with rolling. Live – steam is applied to whole grain in a conditioner. A holding period may be used. A more uniform product with some fines can be produced in a roller mill steam conditioning. The steamed grains are more palatable and preferred by many farmers.

Pelleting

Pellets are collected into mass of feeds formed by expulsion of individual ingredients or mixtures by compacting and forcing through die – openings by mechanical process. There could be two types of pellets :

a) **Hard type:** Pellets are produced on equipment using a combination of rollers and die for pressure and forming. The basic principle is, as the following:

1. All the ingredients are ground and blended together into a pelleting chamber and distributed by means of gravity, centrifugal force and mechanical deflectors.
2. Pressure resulting from rotation of dies and rollers, forces feed through perforations in die, which compresses and forms feed into pellet.
3. Adjustable knives cut pellets into desired length.
4. The pellets are then cooled and dried before bagging or binning (Fig. 4).

b) **Soft type:** These pellets contain over 30 % molasses, are produced in an equipment using a combination of auger and die for pressure and pellet forming. The basic principle of this type of pellet is as following –

   i. A blended mash and molasses is introduced into auger.
   ii. A rotating auger conveys material to the die and builds up pressure for extrusion (expulsion).

iii. Pressure resulting from rotating auger, forces feed through perforations in the die, compressing and forming it into pellets.

iv. Pellets are usually allowed to break off by force of gravity. Sizing is generally random and further handling removes excessively long particles.

v. Pellets are dusted with bentonite or finely ground cotton – seed meal to absorb excess molasses, which would otherwise cause pellets to stick together.

vi. The pellets are cooled and dried before bagging or binning (Fig. 5).

Crumbles

For the production of smaller feed particles, its desirable to use the crumbling process. In this process, pellets are ground on corrugated – rolls and resultant product is graded by sieving over appropriate screen sizes. These days, most of the crumbling mills consist of one pair of corrugated rollers mounted in a frame directly below the cooler. This eliminates the need for additional feeding mechanisms as the pellets are discharged from the cooler. Some of the crumbles are equipped with manually operated by – valves to be used for production of pellets. This reduces the need of changing roll – settings, when changing from crumbles to pellets.

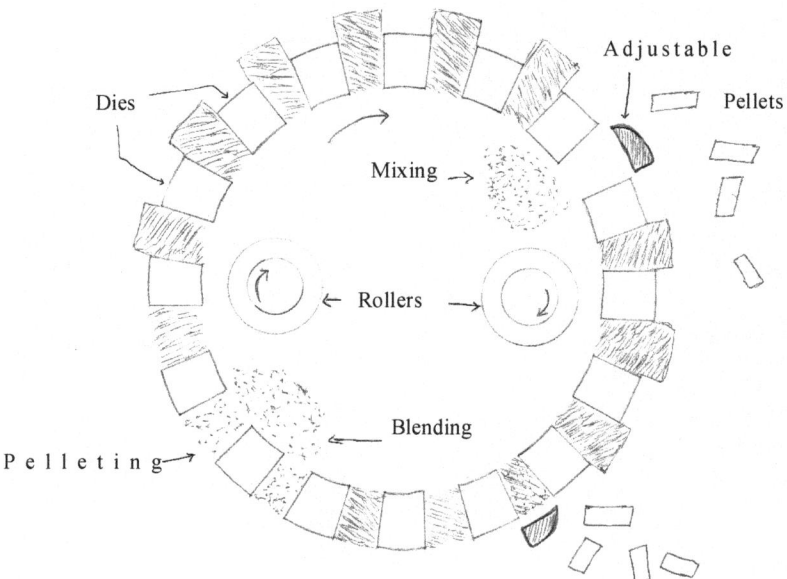

Fig. 4 : Hard Type Pelleting Machine [Diagrammatic Representation] (Cross section)

Extrusion

Such feeds are prepared by passing the grain through a machine with a spiral, tapered screw. In the process, the grain is ground and heated, producing a ribbon – like product. Extrusion cooking has become an important part of the feed industry, for example –

- Gelatinization of cereals
- Feeds for animals.
- Cooking of Soybeans and pulses (for destruction of anti – nutritional factors).
- Cooking of meat meal, fish meal, feather meal et cetra.

Gelatinization of starch

There is complete rupture of the starch granules, which is carried out by a combination of moisture, heat and pressure. There are two advantages :

a) Gelatinization increases the ability of starch to absorb large quantities of water and this leads to improved digestibility and therefore, improved feed conversion.

b) Gelatinization increases the activity at which enzymes (for example, amylase) can break down the linkages of starch, thus converting starch into simpler soluble sugars.

There are two types of 'Extrusion – cookers' :

i) **High temperature extrusion** for short time: In this method, a uniform application of moisture as well as an extruder assembly is designed to work the moisture cereal or cereal mixture into a dough at modest temperature 90°C. A means of elevating the temperature of the dough in the extruder during a very short period of time (15 seconds) to a desired higher temperature of 150°C, within which, the gelatinization becomes relatively complete, the forming of the gelatinized dough into the desired shape by use of a final die and method of cutting the expanded dough into segments of desired length.

ii) **Pressure cooking extruders:** In this method, cereal or cereal mixtures are fed into a pressure – chamber, where steam is applied at 60 lb pressure. Gelatinization is done within 10 minutes at 150°C.

Popping

Popped corn is produced by dry heat, causing a sudden expansion of the grain (for example, pop corn), which actually ruptures the endosperm. During this process, dry-grain is exposed to hot air (about 400°C) for 15-30 seconds. The moisture in the grain turns to steam and causes the kernel to pop-up. The product is usually rolled to reduce bulk and this process increases rumen starch utilization.

Micronizing

The grain is heated to 150°C and then dropped into rolls, which have **spiral grooves** that place diagonal and parallel pressure on the kernels. The product usually resembles steam-flaked grain.

Roasting

This is carried out by passing the grain through a flame (at 150°C) resulting to some expansion of the grains, which produces a palatable product, for example, in Soybeans, Trypsin inhibitor is destroyed and hence, there is improvement in the nutritive value for non-ruminants.

Steam-rolled flakes

Such grains are used partly to kill weed-seeds. This is done by passing steam-up through a tower above a roller-mill. Grains are exposed to steam for a short time (3-5 minutes) before rolling.

Steam-flakes

These are prepared with relatively rigid quality controls where a bigger conditioning chamber is required than for regular steam – rolling. Grain is exposed to high moisture steam for sufficient time (15-30 minutes) to raise the water content to 18-20 % and the grain is then rolled to produce a flat – flake. Such process allows more efficient rupture of starch – granules and produces a more desirable physical texture, for example, the grains - corn, barley; sorghum may have variation due to difference in starches.

Cubed roughages

In this process, dry hay is forced through dies that produce a square product of different hardness. Grinding before cubing is not required but generally water is sprayed on dry hay prior to cubing. Alfa alfa hay produces good cubes which are less likely to break up than grass hays. They show satisfactory performance in cattle as well as facilitate in transportation, handling and feeding.

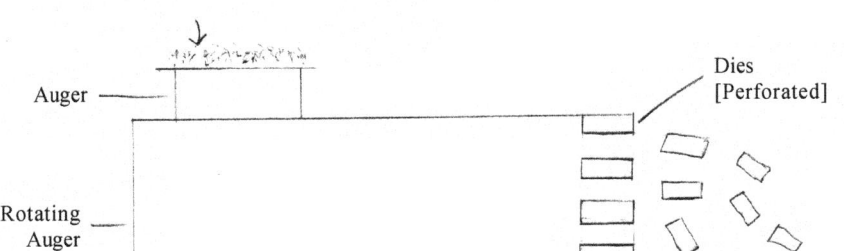

Fig. 5 : Soft Type Pellet Machine [Diagramatic Representation]

Feed mixing

The most important operation in a feed mill is mixing. Actually, this is the single operation that defines the plant as a feed mill. The purpose of such feed mill is to blend together two or more ingredients. There are three types of mixers – vertical, horizontal and continuous.

- a) **Vertical screw type mixer :** This is used in thousands of feed mills. Such mills may have two vertical screw mixers for elevating material. Some mixers have single vertical screw, which are less expensive and show good performance of mixing most ingredients. These mixers are relatively slower than 'Horizontal' mixers and are not generally used in large feed mills.

- b) **Horizontal mixer :** These are also most widely used for large feed mills which have left and right augers. They convey the feed from one end of the mixer to other, while it is tumbled within the mixer. These mixers are frequently equipped with openings at several places along the bottom to help in more discharge. Because material may be difficult to remove from the bottom of a mixer, it is frequently made with a bottom which opens along the entire length. It may be cleaned in other ways, such as by use of air blowing the last material out of the mixer. There are two major advantages of this type of mixer as compared to the vertical mixer –

    i) A shorter mixing cycle, and

    ii) Liquid feed may be added at higher levels.

Such mixers are frequently used where up to 5 % molasses or fat is added in the mixer.

Feed Technology

c) **Continuous mixer :** These are used for mixing higher levels of molasses. One or two shafts with paddles are attached, which convey material from the inlet to the outlet end. The material is conveyed through the mixer and mixed by the paddles. These mixers may be used for adding molasses at the levels of up to 30-40 %. If the molasses is little warmed before being added, it is easier to mix. If it is not mixed, then the mixer shaft generally must operate at much higher speeds.

Feed Blocks

Feed industry has the machines developed to manufacture mineral and protein blocks and these have been designed on the basis of one or two processes incorporating a singular press or a continous extruded principle.

Process : In one of the most exacting operations in the feed mill, a force of about 100 tons is commonly employed to form a block in the **moulding chamber** of the block machine. In order to form a block completely of a specified weight and dimension from a mixed meal, the block machine makes one complete cycle during which time, the following occurs :

1. The door or gate to the moulding chamber is closed and secured automatically.
2. An automatic feed scale, which is an integral part of this machine, charges the press with an exact weight of meal.
3. A hydraulic plunger which may have a seven inch or larger bore is incited to action to travel through its stroke to force all feed into the moulding chamber.
4. High pressure is maintained on the feed in the moulding chamber for a pre – set length of time (retention time) usually 8 seconds.
5. The plunger retracts and the moulding chamber door or gate is automatically opened.
6. The block is ejected onto the packaging table or onto a conveyor for movement to this table.
7. Again the automatic feed scale is tripped and the blocking cycle repeated.
8. Most block machines will continue to cycle automatically, but can be controlled manually to facilitate starting the cycle, testing the pressure and retention time on the block or for ending the blocking cycle.

Equipment

There are several arrangements for a successful blocking operation. One such system would include the following :

1. **The block ingredients are mixed** dry in a mixer and conveyed to a holding bin (above the block press).

2. A variable speed feeder is installed below this holding bin to feed a constant flow of dry meal to a high speed mixer. Steam and liquids are proportional and mixed into the dry meal in this high speed mixer.
3. The mixer discharges into a heavy duty, one or two ton mixer which acts as a conditioner. This mixer, operating continually, feeds the automatic scale, which charges the block press. This conditioner mixer may not be required on all operations, if a homogenous blend is discharged from the blender and if no block quality problems are evidenced.
4. The block machine presses the block and discharges it to a conveyor or to a discharge tube.
5. A box inserter can be used to guide the block into a carton.
6. A **"tape shooter"** is an efficient method of attaching labels to blocks, not boxed or to boxes. However, this necessitates having all labels printed on gummed block tape rolls.
7. Pelletization: Unboxed protein blocks are normally stacked on the side to assure that pressure is applied to the label. Boxed blocks may be stacked on end to assure the sealing of glued or taped box ends.

Formula feed industry

Feed is the largest single item of expense in the production of milk, meat and eggs accounting for about 70 % of total costs. The challenge facing the industry is to formulate, manufacture and distribute feeds that will enable livestock and poultry farmers to produce quality products at the lowest possible cost. In formulating the most efficient and economical ration for livestock and poultry, nutritionists must select ingredients that will supply basic animal requirement for energy, protein, minerals and vitamins. Drugs and other additives are added to fill specific needs.

Manufacturing practices: The first step in producing and marketing a formula feed is calculating a formula based on scientific research that can be produced economically enough to fill a customer's needs. The nutritionist often makes use of a computer to formulate feeds having certain desired nutritional qualities at the least cost of ingredients. Formulation is co-operative effort between nutrition, sales, production and management, however many other factors other than nutrition can affect the success of a feed product on the market.

There are four kinds of feed-complete, supplement or concentrate, base-mixture or super-concentrate and pre-mix. The common forms of commercial formula feed produced are-meals (also called mash), crumbles, pellets (also called cubes), blocks as well as liquid feeds. Feed stuffs are comparative with regard to other commodities in the regulatory scene. Selling by – products and feeds of poor or varying quality gave the industry a bad start. Laws passed to control the sale of ingredients and formula feeds to involve reality regarding dishonest dealings and created an unfavourable image that the industry is still trying to overcome.

Chapter 15

Feeds for Sick and Old Animals

Patients are unable to consume foods and fluids orally when they are suffering from illness. Under surgical conditions, severe burns, severe infectious neonatal infants, congenital anomalies, anorexia, coma or dysfunction of elementary tract etc., special feeding methods should be used for feeding such patients.

Objectives

- To provide water and electrolytes to prevent dehydration and correct electrolyte imbalance.
- To make up the loss of tissue protein.
- To provide energy to meet the daily needs of the patients.

The nutrients used in intravenous feeding are :

a) **Water and electrolytes :** The daily minimum water requirement of an adult on an average is 1.5 liters. Additional water will be required to correct dehydration that might have occurred before therapy. The water loss made up in about 24 hour and the urinary excretion restored to about 300-400 ml in every 8 hrs.

b) **Carbohydrates and alcohol :** Glucose, Fructose and Sorbitol are used in intravenous feeding. Three per cent alcohol @ 8 g/h can also be given; because this provides 7.1 kcal energy / g. Glucose is usually administered as 5 % solution. Fructose is preferred to Glucose, as it can be administered at a concentration of 10-15 % without any adverse effect.

c) **Amino acids :** Solution form of Protein hydrolysates, Synthetic amino acid mixture and a mixture of L-amino acids are available for intravenous feeding. Protein hydrolysates prepared from casein, free from peptides and fortified with Tryptophan are commonly used for intravenous therapy.

d) **Whole blood or plasma :** One litre of whole blood provides about 180 gm proteins including haemoglobin. Blood is used mainly to combat circulatory failure and loss of blood from body. One liter of plasma contain about 60-70 gm of protein. Plasma infusion is given as a measure for increasing plasma protein level when it is low.

e) Vitamins: All the vitamins (twice daily requirements) should be added to intravenous fluid to meet the daily needs of the patient.

Methodology of parental feeding

- Peripheral venous infusion: The needle is inserted in the upper limb veins. It is suitable for giving isotonic solution of Glucose, Saline or other electrolytes for a short period.
- Infusion through **polypropylene** tubes inserted deep into superior or inferior vena cava. It is ideal for long-term parental nutrition and for hypertonic solutions.

Administration of the solutions

a) Weighing the patient and then calculating the fluid needs for 24 hrs
b) Calculating the calorie and nutrient requirements based on body weight.
c) Administrating the fluids initially at a slow rate and then at a rate achieving 3000-3500 ml solution per 24 hrs.
d) Monitoring the potential feeding routine-wise.

Monitoring the feeding regimens

Daily basis: Body weight, fluid balance, blood count, urea, electrolytes, blood glucose, urine & plasma osmo-larity, acid base status, urine electrolyte and nitrogen losses.

Thrice weekly: Serum calcium, Magnesium, Phosphates, Plasma proteins and liver function test clotting studies.

Ten days: Serum B_{12}, Folic acid, Iron, Lactate, Triglyceride and trace elements.

Chapter 16

Pet Animal Nutrition

Dog Feeding

In Asia, dogs are the main pet animal kept both by urban and rural families. They are very versatile and adopt to common food habbits of their masters. Most often, they are fed on the home cooked foods – bread, rice, vegetables, pulses, milk and non – vegetarian meals. Many processed pet foods are also available in the market in the form of "Dry biscuits" or in "Canned form", which provide all the requirements for Energy, Protein, Vitamins, Minerals and some moisture. Like any other farm animal, dogs also require these nutrients for their maintenance and productive purposes like – Growth, Lactation, Gestation, draft [sledge – cart on the ice] etcetra. Dogs and humans have been companions from time immemorial and the **first readymade dog food** was marketed under the name - **DOG CHOW CHEKER** in the year **1926**. Since then such dog – foods have gained popularity. Most of the dog foods are manufactured abroad and marketed in India by Multi – National Companies (MNCs). Following are the guide – lines for feeding :

1. Energy sources: Cereal grains - Jowar, Bajra, Oat, Maize, Sorghum. Average requirement of energy 3000 k.cal / kg of feed.
2. Protein sources: Vegetative origin : very poor in Essential Amino acids. e.g. Soybean, grams, peas [green proteins], beans, other legumes.
3. Fat: 10 % (oil seeds are good sources Protein as well as Fats).
4. Non – starch fibrous feeds (5 %): To tone – up Alimentary canal.
5. Feed supplements: Additional nutrients: Green vegetables (carotenoids), fruits, skimmed milk, curd, butter – milk.
6. Feed Additives: These are Non-nutrients: Mushroom, herbal preparations [no side effects by Aanwala, Aloe-veera].

Neutraceuticals

a) Pre – biotics: Non – digestible food ingredients, which beneficially stimulate Growth / Acivity of Colon – microbes & therefore, improve health, eg. Oligosaccharides.

b) Pro-biotics: Living microbial cultures, eg. Lactobacillus (curd), Streptococcus. These are the food for (a).

c) Syn – biotics: Combination of above both, eg. Enzymes, Salmonella.

[Palatability (taste): 3 basic factors increase palatability : Flavour, Aroma, Physical characteristics (eg. Softness due to some moisture, Crunchiness, Chewiness)].

Nurient % ages

Species	Protein	Carbohydrate	Fat	Fibre
Dog	20	60	10	Not essential
Cat	30	Not essential	25	Not essential

Types of Dog food

1. Dry food : [< than 10 % moisture], (a) Vegetative: Whole cereal grains or cereal-by products [Wheat middling, wheat germ meal, corn gluten meal, soybean meal, soya grits]. (b) Animal Products: Meat / meat-meal / meat by products, bone or bone meal / Poultry products / dried skimmed milk (milk fat is removed after centrifugation) / dried whey [liquid left after separation of casein etc. during cheese making]. (c) Commercial: Feed meal, pellets, biscuits, kibbles (broken biscuits), extruded or flakes.

2. Semi – moist food: Moderate moisture (25 %). Such feeds are protected against spoilage without refrigeration by their content of sucrose, propylene glycol & sorbates. They commonly contain Animal products, eg. Meat or its by products, Fish or its by products, chicken or it by products, Milk precuts (eg. Cheese), Fats & Oils [eg. Lard (of swine), Tallow (of cattle), Soybean meal, Soy flour, Vitamins & minerals].

3. Canned food: High in moisture (75 %). Such feeds are formulated to be nutritionally complete [that is, low meat / meat by products.

4. Frozen food: Very high meat ingradients & moisture, longer shelf – life (keeping quality, as it can be refrigerated), Thawed (melted) food is soft + dental care is taken.

Nutritional Care of Orphans

Technically, an orphan is any young animal that does not have access to the milk or care of its mother. Circumstances that may render young puppy or kitten orphans include :

- The death of dam.
- The production of an inadequate quantity or quality of milk.
- Or, rejection of the young by the dam.

Whatever the underlying cause, once puppies or kittens are orphaned, they depend on humans for the provision of maternal care, proper nutrition, & a suitable environment. Although it is difficult, if not impossible, to fully compensate for the absence of the dam, the use of proper management & feeding techniques can result in the development of normal, healthy puppies & kittens.

Proper room temperature for orphan puppies & kittens:

Age (wks)	Temperature
0-1	85-90°F
2-4	80-85°F
5-6	70-75°F
> 6	70°F.

Practical feeding management

- Provide a warm & clean environment that is free from draft (dust).
- Feed a commercial milk replacer.
- Estimate correct amount of formula based on the animal's age & weight.
- Divide the formula into 4-5 equal feedings / d.
- Bottle feed or use a feeding tube.
- Weigh them periodically.
- Introduce semi – solid food at 3 wks.
- Wean to dry pet food by 6 to 10 wk.

Cat Feeding

Cat is carnivore that has evolved to a diet which is :

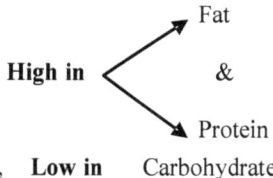

High in Fat & Protein

But, **Low in** Carbohydrate

Cat is dependent on a supply of at least some animal derived food stuff in its diet. It has no characteristic type of metabolism that is, it has atypical metabolism. Due to such dependency on animal origin food, it is regarded as an **Obligate Carnivore** (dog is omnivorous, that is, not binding, optional). Therefore, the interesting aspect is that, the requirement is adjusted accordingly, that is, not characteristic for Tom (father) or Queen (mother). Generally, cats being carnivorous, its normal diet consist of meat, which is rich in **TAURINE** and thus, take care of taurine requirements. The problem arises when the commercial diets comprising of cereal and grains are fed to these animals, because **plants are poor sources of Sulfur amino acids.**

Kitten Feeding

Kittens at birth, usually weigh about 100 g and they are entirely dependent on their mother's (queen's) milk, for about 4 wks.

By 5th wk : They begin to eat adult food and would start to eat finally minced or chopped moist food.

By 7-8 wks : The total nutrient intake coming from supplementary food, which should be at least about 70-80 %. A weaning kitten at this stage, weighs about 800 g.

A growing kitten requires about 200 k. cal ME / kg.

By 6 mo of age : Kitten grow rapidly and attain adult weight around 3.5 kg.

By one year of age : They settle down to an average adult intake of 90 k.cal / kg.

Adult Cat feeding

Wild : Cat is an opportunist. They eat as and when they catch and kill prey. Therefore, their feeding habits are irregular.

Domestic Cats : They nurture on palatable foods, prefer to eat many small meals, about 15 per day (rather than one or two). The average pet-cat can weigh about 4 kgs and needs about 350 k.cal per day, through 100 g dry food.

Female Gestation requirements: This is about 4 times her normal maintenance needs.

Chapter 17

Principles of Zoo Mammal Nutrition

Feeding wild animals in captivity presents a fearful challenge. There are hundreds of species to consider, each representing millions of years of evolutionary adaptation to particular ecological system.

Natural foods range from Ants to Antelopes. (Antelope = African (deer like) ruminant, for example - gazelles, gnus, kudus and impala) and **Mouth structures** vary from Edentate (toothless) to Carnassial (specialized pre-molars and molars).

Natural feeding & foraging strategies include
- a) Fossorial (animals adapted for digging).
- b) Terrestrial (animals living on earth or ground).
- c) Arboreal (animals living on trees).
- d) Aquatic types. (animals living in or near water).

Stomach : These may be
- a) Single
- b) Quadruple.

Intestines: These may be
- a) Tube like or
- b) Equipped with a caecal fermentation vat (vat = large vessel).

On the surface, the problem appears unsolvable, & it certainly is not easy. But the need persists to nourish all captive species as appropriately as possible & it is not feasible to wait until a **DATA BASE** is developed comparable with that which exists for domestic animals. Actually domestic animal data can be very useful for the estimation of nutrient needs of wild counterparts.

2(a) A useful strategy for formulating diets for **Captive Wild animals** is to consider :
- i) **Dietary habbits** in the wild.
- ii) Oral & Gastric Intestinal **Morphology.**

iii) Needs of **Similar species**, whose requirements are known.

iv) Cage or enclosure **environment** of the Captive animal.

Natural food provide **CLUES**

a) As to Nutrient Intake and

b) Whether diets in the wild have low / high amounts of certain nutrients, such as **Fibre** or **Secondary metabolites** which may influence :

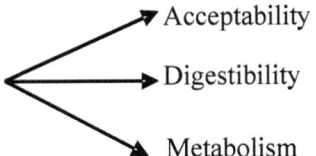

Acceptability
Digestibility
Metabolism

Although Oral Anatomy, Morphology of G.I.T. usually correlate with natural diet, the **Giant Panda** represents an interesting exception due to following –

a) a Carnivore like **Jaw**.

b) **Teeth** more suited for Crushing [than Shearing i.e. Tearing apart].

c) No capability for lateral Grinding.

All the above are characteristics of PANDA. Its natural diet consists pre – dominantly of **Fibrous BAMBOO**, yet its GUT is a rather Simple Tube, limiting the fermentation of such food.

2(b) In most cases, though, Mouth Structures, such as :

- Lip shape
- Dentition

help define the type of food an animal can most easily ingest & chew.

For example,

Black Rhinoceros

This has a **Pre – hensile** (capable of grasping) **Upper Lip** that is well designed for Browsing & **lack of Incisors** makes Grazing difficult. On the other hand,

Hippopotamus

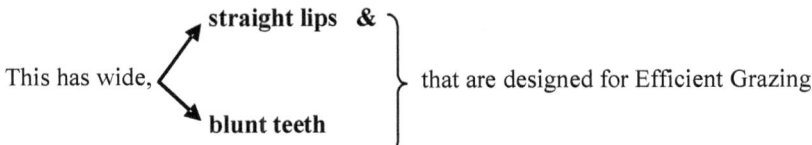

This has wide, straight lips & blunt teeth that are designed for Efficient Grazing.

2(c) The presence of a **RUMINO – RETICULUM** suggests that the animal's Quantitative requirements are similar to those of **CATTLE & SHEEP**, & that there is significant MICROBIAL synthesis of the **Vitamin 'B' complex** & **Vitamin K**.

If the animal's gut has a **CAECUM & COLON** that are capacious enough to support Microbial Fermentation, its nutrient needs are likely to be similar to those of HORSE.

A simple stomach with limited space in the lower gut, for Microbial activity is similar to that of **Swine.**

Thus, one might extrapolate NUTRIENT REQUIREMENTS from domestic species with known needs to WILD SPECIES, that are SIMILAR in :
- Dietary habbits and
- GIT structure & function.

The dimensions of the SPACE in which animals are confined will influence their ENERGY REQUIREMENTS & Food items growing in that environment will affect the need for supplemental food.

Nutrient Requirements

The Basic Needs of all **Vertibrate** tissues appear to be nearly the same:

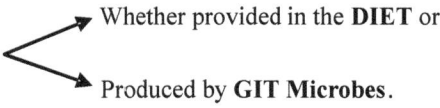

Whether provided in the **DIET** or

Produced by **GIT Microbes**.

Chapter 18

Feeding Zoo and Wild Animals

Carnivore [Carnivora]
Members of this family are mostly **flesh-eaters** and share features that show **hunting lifestyle**.

Limbs: These are very powerful, agile quick moving, very active.

Forward-facing eyes: These help in judging distance accurately.

Teeth: All have very strong canine teeth for cutting.

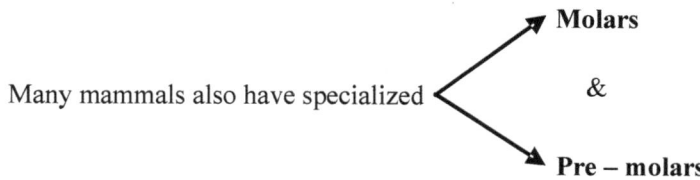

Many mammals also have specialized Molars & Pre – molars

These molars & pre-molars function like **shears** to slice through flesh (meat).

One exception is the **Giant Panda**, which is almost-entirely **Herbivore**, although, most other members of carnivora family would supplement their diet with Vegetation, when necessary.

Pinnipeds [Marine mammals]
In some systems of classification, Pinnipeds are considered as members of Carnivora, for example, marine mammal – Elephant Seal.

Most pinnipeds are collected from isolated island rookeries, shoelines or seaice. Use of a so – called "Wally" net is the most efficient means of collecting large Seals, such as above Elephant seal. Large transport - cage carries such big animal to shore.

Felids [Felidae]
Both domestic and wild cats have always fascinated humankind. Non – domestic felids are popular zoo exhibits and it is the rare zoo that does not show one or more species (there are fourty). They vary in size from a Sand cat (weighing 2 kg) to a Siberian tiger (weighing over 300 kgs).

Feeding and Nutrition

Although a number of commercial Carnivore or Felid diets are available abroad (eg. U.S. & Canada), but fact is that, a few cats refuse to eat the prepared diets. Some zoos or private owners do not prefer commercial diets for their animals. **Because, the ideal diet would be whole animals of a size proportionate to normal prey**. Such a diet is not only impractical, but also unacceptable to public.

Small rodents, rabbits and poultry may be fed to smaller felids. **Chicken necks and backs** are often fed, but are totally inadequate nutritionally. Although ash content of chicken necks is over 50 %, therefore mineral intake is high. Energy and protein intake is insufficient.

Meat, heart, liver and kidney are severely deficient in Calcium and have a poor Ca : P ratio, making them unsuitable as foods without heavy supplementation.

Thumb rule (for quantities of feed intake):

Moderate cat may require	5 % of body weight.
A 300 kg tiger may require	8 % of body weight.
Young growing cat may require	25 % of body weight.
At Gestation stage, cat may require	30 % of body weight.

[if feeding a large offspring (litter), then a cat's requirement is increased to 50 % of body].

Therefore, all zoo animals should be fed according to the individual needs of each animal at a particular growth stage based on weight gain / loss. Most felids have adapted to a **"Feast-or-famine"** routine. In the wild, a cat may not eat everyday (particularly after engorgement). Some zoos fast their cats one day each week on the reason that this is natural for cats and therefore, beneficial.

Feeding records

This is important, that is, food consumption should be monitored, but this may be difficult with **"Pride of Lions"**. Felids have some unusual dietary requirements. Protein requirement is almost double that of Canids (for example dogs, foxes, wolves). Also, Felids are unable to convert Carotene to Vitamin A. Therefore, they must be provided with pre-formed Vitamin A.

Herbivores

Elephant [Proboscidea]

In the wild, a mature Asian - African elephant will spend as many as 18 hrs feeding / d, eating as much as 300 kg of feed. This food is high in fibre but, low in other nutrients.

A typical diet for an adult per day:

2 kg	=	Oats
23 kg	=	Lettuce [succulent salad leaf]
23 kg	=	Carrots
200 gm	=	Mineral – Vitamin + salt (rock) supplement.
300 gm	=	Ferrous sulphate [If housed on cement than earth]

Normally, food passage through the elephant's digestive tract takes 35 hrs. Some concentrated pelleted feeds may also be included, because elephants are not quite efficient in digesting hay. Behavioral requirements suggest balancing roughage and concentrate. They take 200 litres of water per day in one or two receiving.

Horse, Ass, Zebra [Equide]

A wild horse weighs 300 kg on an average. A wild Asian - African ass is similar to domestic donkey. Anatomically, Zebras appear to be a compromise between horse and ass. The major difference is in their colouration.

Feeding and Nutrition of horses: Pelleted horse feed containg 12 % protein, 1 kg pellets per 100 kg body weight plus high fibre hay of equal amounts, makes a good ration.

Blocks of both mineralized and plain salt would be required on some surface away from moisture. Otherwise, mineral would run – off to surrounding soil. In cold weather, energy requirement increases. Protein requirement enhances in productive animals-Young foals, Gestation / lactating mares. One feeder of one meter length per two animals and two such feeders per unit are generally ideal for feeding the horses.

Rhinoceros [Rhinocerotidae]

There is no problem with horn (s), if broken. Because, there is no real skeletal – support. Therefore, **re – growth** begins immediately. [In cattle calf, dehorning is done withing 10 d, because horn – buttons are not formed in the skull].

There are three types of Rhinoceros as following :

a) Indian
b) Black: are browsers (like goats) and have prehensile tip on the upper lip capable of grasping feed.
c) White: This type is a grazer (like cattle), characterized by a long head and square lips. The digestive system is similar to that in Eqine.

Territorial behavior

Black one is temperamental i.e. indifferent, the whole of natural tendencies are determined by its physical constitution:

i) Their behavior would indicate serve myopia, but excellent hearing (good olfactory senses), because of their habit of returning to chosen spots. This act is shown or accomplished by a **Scraping motion with their back feet**.

ii) They urinate at some **localized areas**. These areas once established, are almost impossible to change.

Feeding and Nutriton

The Indian and black rhinos, both are browsers. The Indian Rhino, with its long, sharp lower incisors, is especially capable of cutting branches and saplings (juicy plants) upto five centimeters. Lacking browse, both of these species, as well as the Square-lipped Rhino, i.e. White, depend on most mixtures of hay and grain. Pelleted horse feeds are readily accepted by all three species. Hay is required to be of good quality, but a diet of fine alpha – alpha hay, often proves to have too laxative an effect. On coarse hay, the Indian Rhino tends to develop stomach upset, but this can easily be corrected by the addition of oats, bran, yams (a tuber), carrots or greens. Total daily intake for an adult animal weighing 2500 kg would be 40 kg dry matter. An individual may drink 200 litres of water in twenty four hour period. Horn length of African Rhino limits the depth, the animal can reach.

Hippopotamus (Hippopotamidae)

A typical diet for an adult Hippopotamus would comprise :

50 kg	=	Hay
5 kg	=	Cattle grazing pellets (14 %)
3 loaves	=	Bread
10 kgs	=	Potatoes, cabbage, carrots, apples & onions

+ Fresh grass (greatly relished, but should be introduced carefully to avoid digestive upsets).

Camel [Camelid] : A pseudo-ruminant

- All South American Camelids (S.A.C.) are basically grazers, but also browsers.
- Grasses in their native countries are usually low in protein (5 %) Even though they can subsist on such poor forage, these animals will do better on a mixed **Grass – legume pasture**.

- **Alpha – alpha pasture:** Its not advisable to graze these animals straight on such feed. Although **Tympanitis** is uncommon, it may occur. There is no danger of Bloat from feeding this pasture. In fact, this feed would be the most desirable dry forage. Grass hays are acceptable, if they are of good quality (12 %).
- **Intake**

An adult with activity (this may increase)   = 2 %
Gestation / Lactating & / growing juvenile   = 4 %
Llamas that are packing   = should receive concentrate.

[Llamas are known to be affected with White muscle disease. Protection against this disease requires Periodical injections of **Vitamin E + Selenium**]

- Old World Camelids: Dromedary and Bactrian camels, for example, are adaptable in eating habbits. Both are domestic species. In their native habitat, they both browse and graze.
- In zoos, they prosper on good quality Alpha – alpha or Oat hay. Animals heavily used for camel rides should be supplemented with concentrates.

Deer [Cervidae]

Following may be considered for feeding :

- Cervids are true ruminants and therefore, herbivores. They feed on grass, twigs, leaves, bark and young shoots of trees and other plants.
- In Captivity, deer would usually browse on the existing grasses, branches and twigs in large deer parks.
- However, the existing vegetation would soon be destroyed unless supplemental browse and grain are provided.
- They prefer alpha – alpha or clover (berseem) hay. All hay should be fed in racks or mangers.
- In small enclosures, freshly cut browse can be tied in bundles and hung up.
- Grain should also be provided in feeding boxes, especially in the colder months.
- Commercially available Dairy Chow and herbivore pellets are excellent in this case.
- Pellets of various sizes have been provided, depending upon the species involved and the management process.
- Salt blocks and mineral blocks should be available all the time.
- Good quality hay are essential for good production and management.

Chapter 19

Palo Podrido Feed

The bio-degradation process dates back to time immemorial when some wild ruminant animals were spotted feeding on the tree –woods in South Chile. The natives of this place called this feed as **"*Palo Podrido* (Huempe)"**, meaning – 'animal feed', as opined by **F. Zadrazil** of Germany. Later on, it was found that this wood was actually degraded by certain types of fungi under natural conditions and decomposed to Spent-wood, which turned out to be the animal feed. The scientists started working on these fungi as well as this type of process. Lately, the fungi were found to be belonging to higher basidiomycetes class, called: **White-rot-fungi**. They mainly degraded lignin of the wood, however cellulose and hemicelluloses to a limited extent only.

But, surprisingly it was found that the digestibility and crude protein content increased to a considerable extent. Later on, the scientists started working on spent-straws too. The cereal straws (lignocellulosics) constituted a staple-feed (basal) in the developing countries for these ruminant animals. But, the presence of lignin (a biological plastic) limits the utilization of these cereal straws in the rumen eco-system. Thus, the concept of Solid State Fermentation (SSF) sparked into this type of investigation. Some examples of such white-rot-fungi were: *Pleurotus ostreatus, Coprinus cineus, Sporotrichum thermophile, Phanerochaete chrysosporium, Polyporous berkeleyi, Neurospora crssa, Alternaria tenius* to name a few. Some examples of substrates upon which such types of fungi grew for SSF were: wheat straw, paddy straw, paddy husks, ground nut shells, sugarcane bagasse, barley straw, sunflower stalk, aspen wood, birch wood, saw dust etc. The resurgence of interest in the use of straw from cereal and grain crops as animal feed had been witnessed in early nineties to maintain the performance of animals. Following were some of the variations undertaken by different scientific groups:

- Specially designed extruders, pneumatic cyclones and disk refiner for allowing intimate contact of straw particles with the chemicals. Such treatment decomposed the lignin moiety of the cohesive ligno –cellulosic complex. But, the treatment dictated certain limitations – the higher concentrations of chemicals were required under pressure for better efficiency, huge quantity of water was used for washing out the chemicals, loss due to higher moisture content, generation of effluent and consequently, high expenses on waste – management (otherwise environmental pollution).

- Decomposition of plant residues by pure cultures of thermophilic moulds was also studied and a lot of variation was observed. Since it was very difficult at that stage, to come to a conclusion about the degradability of lignin by these moulds based on the data, it had been strongly felt a need for the simple and sensitive assay.

- Yet in another study, estimations were carried out without the use of chemicals (for example, sulphuric acid), it was found that, about 5 % methoxyl in the lignin isolated from legumes and about 10 % methoxyl in lignin isolated from various grasses and very little difference was found in the methoxyl content of the lignin isolated from the corresponding faeces, which indicated that there was very little breakdown of these linkages in the lignin molecule during passage through digestive tract.

- Softwood lignin and lignifications were investigated. Alkali treatment did not decrease methoxyl content of lignin. High carbohydrate content accounted for the lower value of methoxyl groups in the lignin preparation.

- Further studies on lignin and lignifications were undertaken for the comparative evaluation of native lignins, for characterization of enzymatically liberated hard – wood lignins as well as isolation and characterization of bagasse native lignin.

- Growth studies with *Streptomyces* cultures were studied and production of pigments in the Asparagine – glucose – agar and Tyrosine – glucose – agar media were tested. After 10 d growth at 37°C, the plates were observed and score was based on visual relative examination.

- Microbes were studied in cattle fed with a constant ration and a culture medium was developed for carbon source – inoculation of mixed anaerobes having a mixed gas atmosphere of CO_2 and N_2 (85 : 15).

- Activity of aromatic alcohol oxidase was studied in the growth medium of *Polysticus versicular*, unraveling the direct involvement of enzymes.

- Enzymatic degradation of soft – wood lignin was studied by white – rot – fungi and possibility of direct role of extracellular and non – specific enzymes was advocated.

- Biodegradation of isomers of Benzene Hexa Chloride (BHC) was studied and faster breakdown under anaerobic condition was observed. It was also reported that repeated addition of chlorinated cyclo hexane insecticide

to flooded soil caused the enrichment of specific microbes resulted in the enhanced degradation of this addition.
- Other works indicated that white – rot – fungi (higher basidiomycetes) could utilize lingnin alongwith cellulose and other components of the substrate.
- Upgrading the straw quality as ruminant feed through biological treatment using Phanerochaete chrysosporium (a white – rot – fungus) was also studied. Increasing the lignolytic activity with a minimum loss of associated polysaccharides had been the prime objective of this study.
- Gradually, such type of interesting research area caught the attention of various other groups' world over. In past couple of decades, this research field gained tremendous momentum, so much so that, there was a lot of overlapping of simultaneous work and therefore, great communication among different researchers.

Solid State Fermentation (SSF) Research in the Developing World

The research focussed mainly on *Pleurotus ostreatus* [Commonly known as Oyster mushroom; the French version: CHAMPIGN; (Coprinus species tested for higher temperatures)] and prepared their 'spawn' on un – infected sorghum grains (alternatively, millet or wheat grains were also used by other workers). After thorough cleaning and boiling, these grains were filled in the 250 ml heat-resistant bottles with calcium oxide mixed (1% of grain quantity) and were autoclaved at 15 lb pressure for 20 min. These bottles were then inoculated with the above fungi aseptically in the UV chamber separately and kept for incubation at 25°C for a week. This spawn was used to treat the different straws in the polypropylene bags to **optimize** the different cultural conditions – temperatures, moisture levels, incubation periods, light (in the BOD incubator), supplemental nutrients N and S, buffer concentrations, heat treatments, mineralization as well as composting, other substrates.

The aliquots were analyzed for different attributes – crude protein (CP), neutral detergent fibre (NDF), acid detergent fibre (ADF), hemicelluloses, permanganate – lignin, cellulose, pH, bio – mass, water soluble, *in vitro* dry matter digestibility (IVDMD), digestible dry matter recovery (DDMR) including nylon bag dry matter digestibility (NBDMD). During above fermentation, the CP content increased significantly in general with respect to their corresponding controls possibly due to proportionately lower N – loss compared to C – loss. The carbon loss was found to be due to a loss of cellulose and or hemicellulose. The fungus might have utilized such carbohydrates, resulting in some dry matter loss. These findings reflected that such fungi were known to lack the ability of fixing atmospheric nitrogen and therefore, tend to conserve available nitrogen for their growth. There was no effect of exposure to light in these studies.

There were actually two phases during the colonization of such fungi. In the initial phase of a week-ten days, the fungus used soluble nutrients of the substrates for their own establishment and therefore, there was slow initial increase in digestibility. And thereafter in the final phase, the fungus attacked the fibrous portion of substrate enhancing the digestibility. This was due to weakening of lingo-carbohydrate complexe (the extent of weakening depended mainly on the substrate type and its preferential use by the fungus in question).

The scientists (including the **author**) were more concerned for the fungal growth upto the mycelia-stage only and this took about three to four weeks' time in general and then the further growth was stopped. They did not want 'fruit – body formation' [that is mushroom formation (Champignon)] as it sapped more of the available nutrients. The German scientists thought it a little commercial application. They also worked extensively on optimizing the cultural conditions of different white-rot-fungal species. But, they had profited by dual advantages -on the upper part of the substrates, they grew and harvested edible crop of mushrooms for commercial consumption of human beings and the lower spent -substrates were used as ruminant feed.

Discovery of Ligninase Enzyme: Biotechnological Perpective

In 1983, various laboratories announced the discovery of an extracellular H_2O_2 requiring enzyme in a white-rot fungus : ***Phanerochaete chrysosporium*** that catalyzes lignin degradation in the culture growth medium. The researchers had isolated and purified this enzyme, which was able to degrade lignin model compounds in general and the C-C and ether bond cleavage reactions, in particular. This enzyme, however, was obligatorily depended on the presence of hydrogen peroxide for its activity *in vitro*. Results from various laboratories had also shown that this enzyme was a peroxide type metalloprotein. Further studies revealed that ligninase activity in *P. chrososporium* might be associated with more than one enzyme-isozymes too. The variation in the enzyme sizes may probably due to post-translational modifications, strain differences, cultural conditions and age.

Searching for Genes

Once it was evident that lignin degradation was catalyzed by ligninase, many laboratories tried to isolate the ligninase genes. Rapid advancement in recombinant DNA technology was probed not only to isolate the genes but also to over – produce the ligninase for commercial use. The **CRUX** of the problem lied in the isolation of ligninase genes. By the diligent use of the molecular biological techniques, it might be possible to isolate any gene whose protein product was available. A couple of following techniques to isolate such genes may be tried.

- **Immunoscreening :** This was tried as antigen – antibody reaction. Antibodies were raised against a protein whose gene was identified. Total mRNAs were isolated and full – length cDNAs were cloned in suitable expression vectors and transformed into suitable host such as *E. coli* or yeast. Cells harbouring recombinant DNA were replica plated on to antigen agar. Following the growth, the cells within the colonies were lysed by exposure to chloroform vapour. The antibody was linked to a solid support such as DEM – cellulose filter or PVC support and brought into gentle contact with the lysed cells to allow adsorption of antigen to antibody. This complex was detected by incubating the sheet with the second antibody protein that was radiolabelled. Untreated antibody could be washed away and position of the antigen – antibody complex could be determined by auto radiography, the position of the bacterial cells, which were synthesizing the antigen, on the master petri plate could be identified.

- **Diffential Screening :** For the isolation of genes that were expressed at different stages of life cycle or environmental conditions such as developmentally regulated genes and heat shock genes. Similarly, lignin-modifying genes were expressed in stationary phase and not in exponentially growing cells. Differently expressed genes could be identified by DNA-Hybidization techniques. mRNAs were extracted from exponentially growing and stationary phase cells (lignin expressing and not expressing). Both of these mRNAs were used to synthesize different radioactive cDNA -probes. Each probe was hybridized to identical blots from genomic library or cDNA constructed from ligninase expressing cultures. Since ligninase mRNAs were present only in the induced cells, these genes would be visualized only with the induced probe (and not with the un- induced probe). Therefore, it would be possible to identify ligninase- coding genes using this technique and it was possible to isolate ligninse genes.

Future Projections

Lignocellulosics have the tremendous potential of recycling agricultural wastes into food, feed and fuel. Though, good beginning has been made in understanding the processes underlying the degradation of various crop residues by white- rot fungi, but future researches should address to the aspect of suitability of species for various substrates and in-depth understanding of the enzymology of lignin degradation as well as mode of action. Ideal and optimum interaction between the substrate and white-rot fungi, the kinetic properties of the metabolic processes should also be worked out. This would lead to the production of active ligninase enzyme on commercial scale.

Molecular characterization of the cloned-DNA fragment in plastid containing a new gene engineered for producing desired mutant is important. Therefore, efforts may be made to use mutants of white-rot fungi lacking in cellulose and / or hemicellulase activities during SSF of ligno-carbohydrate crop residues, so that holocellulose may not be degraded, thus reducing the extent of organic matter loss.

Hypothesis

Penetration of fungal – hyphae may take place in these possible ways :
1. The fungus grows in the central cavity – the lumen of the cell and spreads in the neighbouring cells through pores or perforated zones, or
2. The enzymes of fungus facilitate penetration through the cell wall themselves.

    By doing so,
    i) Either lignin is removed, or
    ii) Modified, that is, de-polymerized, but **re-polymerized back** or what !!!
3. Fungus could also degrade modified – lignin, which leads to the concept of bio-leaching (**in that case, re – polymerization may not be possible**).

The discovery of ligninase in 1983 signified for many scientists, the end of a long search for the biological catalysts involved in lignin degradation and start of new bio-technological developments based on the enzyme. However, they had been unable to use the enzyme to degrade lignin with any degree of success. Under these circumstances, they might run a real risk of losing sight of the importance of ligninase to lignin – breakdown and its potential for implementing either in its :

$$\begin{cases} \text{Natural form} \\ \text{Modified or} \\ \text{Mimicked} \end{cases}$$

Accordingly, they suggested three possible areas where, rationalization would contribute greatly to our understanding of how to use the enzyme *in vitro* :

- **First:** How does ligninase attack lignin *in vivo* ? Is the attack made by a mediator, like Veratryl alcohol or direct ?
- **Second:** Where is ligninase located *in vivo*? Is it fixed in space, located on the fungal – hyphae or freely diffusing ?
- **Third:** How is further polymerization of phenolic compounds by ligninase with its attendant inhibitory effects on the enzyme controlled or avoided ?

Chapter 20

Unconventional Feeds

Since hundreds of years, Livestock animals are an integral part of crop – livestock system. In the life style of Indian people, livestock had always been given a special and respectful place and this will continue in the years to come. Despite considerable deficit of feeds, the above may be one of the reasons of steadily increasing livestock production in our country. Almost all assessments made during the past eight decades, have shown deficits of different orders in respect of following for the availability of :

- Dry fodders
- Green fodders and
- Concentrates

Such surprising phenomenon is inviting our attention for reviewing systems of assessment for finding out the status of consumption and the gap between the above. Production of milk, meat, fibre, chicken and egg is increasing, though. Therefore, there is gap between the availability and requirements of different feeds. Because India is facing shortage of both protein and energy rich animal feeds, a large number of agro – forest based unconventional by products have been used. Some of these feeds were found to be promising, while others affected the performance of the animals, due to presence of incriminating factors present in them. But after detoxification, these feeds were suitable for animal feeding. Some of these feeds are :

Feed	Nutritive value		Feeding value
	Protein	Energy	
Kapok (Silk cotton) seed meal	20 % CP	1.30 Mcal ME / kg	May be fed to ruminants. Discoloration of egg yolk. Beyond 10 % depressed growth and feed intake. In poultry, mortality increased.
Kokam cake (Garcinia indica)	9 % DCP	80 % TDN	Crossbred calves – 500 g average daily gain (15 % in concentrate mixture).
Kosum cake (Schleichera leasa)	15 % DCP	80 % TDN	Crossbred calves – 418 g average daily gain, 35 % in concentrate mixture, broilers @ 17 %
Linseed [flax] meal (Linum usitatissimum)	34 % CP	1.60 Mcal ME / kg	Mucilages lead to beak necrosis and exert laxative effect. Contains protective factor against selenosis. Toxic to poultry, if Pyridoxine is not supplemented.
Mango seed kernel cake (Mangifera indica)	6 % DCP	50 % TDN	Milch cows (10 % in concentrate mixture)
Niger seed cake (Guizotia abysainica)	32 % CP	50 % TDN	Crossbred cattle, (57 % in concentrate mixture)
Palm kernel meal (Elaeis quineensis)	20 % CP	1.90 % Mcal ME / kg	Incorporated at 30 % level in poultry diets successfully. Commonly fed to ruminants. Rich in sulphur containing amino acids.
Safflower meal (Carthamum tinctorius), [partially dehulled]	40 % CP	2 Mcal ME / kg	Poor performance in poultry on unhulled meal. Limited usage in grower and layer diets due to high fibre without lysine supplementation.
Sesame meal (Sesamum indicum), [partially dehulled]	40 % CP	2 Mcal ME / kg	15 % in poultry diets with lysine and mineral supplementation.
Spent Annato seeds (Bixa orellama)	8 % DCP	67 % TDN	Crossbred calves – 300 g average daily gain, (20 % in concentrate mixture)
Sunflower meal (Helianthus annus)	36 % CP	2.10 Mcal ME / kg	5 % in poultry diets with lysine supplementation.
Tamarind seed (Tamarindus indicus), [kernel powder, decorticated]	1.3 % DCP	67 % TDN	Calf starter – 728 g average daily gain, bullocks were fed @ 1.5 kg / d without any adverse effects.

Indian subcontinent alone is reported to have at least 86 different oil seed meals. Due to the presence of anti – nutritional factors, high fibre content and poor nutritive value, the utilization of these ingredients is restricted. Most of the work concentrated for feeding these oil meals as such without any suitable and economic detoxification to convert them into a wholesome protein or energy substitutes. A concerted effort to identify the incriminating factors and their cost effective detoxification for easy adoption by farmers and feed compounding industry followed by systematic animal experimentation are needed for better utilization of feed resources.

Concept of Unconventional Feeds

Ruminants and non-ruminants are fed **conventional feeds** like forages, cereals, milling byproducts and oilcakes in animal production system. These feeding systems are mostly practised in the temperate regions, where agriculture is much advanced. In the Asian tropics, agro-industrial byproducts have taken place in the above, which include both the crop residues (paddy straw, wheat straw, stovers etc.) and feeds like sal-seed, rubber-cake, neem-cake and palm-cake.

The term **unconventional** feed or non-conventional feed is a relative term and may differ from country to country, region to region and time to time. Normally such feed refers to the **feed ingredient which has not been used up to now for animal feeding**. For example, paddy straw is conventional feed in India, northern part of Sri Lanka, Bangladesh etc. as it is fed to cattle and buffaloes for centuries. But in Midwestern part of Sri Lanka, southern region of the Philippines, Indonesia etc. it is a unconventional feed as it is not fed to the animals because of the availability of good grasses through pasture and other fodder crops. Such feed is generally organic-it could be bulky like crop residues or concentrated like sal-meal, neem-cake etc.

The agro-industrial byproducts including unconventional feed available are many, which could form a part of livestock feeding system. They may form a part of livestock feeding system and grouped according to their nutrient contents as following –

- **Energy – rich supplements** like molasses from cane, beet, citrus, rejected bananas, pineapple wastes, cassava byproducts;
- **Protein – rich supplements** like oilcakes, fish-meals, meals, pulse peals, animal organic waste (cattle, sheep, pig and poultry manure);
- **Byproducts** which supply mostly the minerals, like bone – meals, seaweeds;
- Miscellaneous byproducts which supply energy and protein – like byproducts from the brewery, fruit, vegetable industries.

Section 02: Applications

Chapter 21

Basic Research
(Development of Bio-methylation Technique)

Gas Chromatography (GC) was discovered in 1954, a very sensitive technique, which paved way to this world for the resolution of the sample leading to detection & identification of the minutest quantity of the desired sample.

Fatty acids were usually converted into corresponding methyl esters (FAME) to improve volatility and to reduce peak tailing for GC. Usually, FAME could be conveniently prepared by heating lipids with a large excess of either acid- or base-catalyzed reagents. Whereas, acid-catalyzed reagents form FAME from both free fatty acids (FFA) and O-acyl lipids base-catalyzed reagents caused only transesterification, i.e. conversion of O-acyl lipids to FAME and do not usually form FAME from FFAs. A base-catalyzed reaction was a useful alternative to acid-catalyzed reactions when a lipid sample contained acid-labile FAs such as propenoids, present in **seed oils** from the Malvales order, such as cottonseed oil. To effect solublization of nonpolar lipids such as triacylglycerols in methanol. the predominant solvent in derivatization reagents, benzene was frequently added to the derivatizalion reaction mixture. However, due to **health concerns**, use of benzene was discouraged. To help solubilize nonpolar lipids, methylene chloride and tetrahydrofuran had been used in place of benzene.

Conventionally, a lipid extract had been used for FAME preparation regardless of transesterification procedure and solubilzing reagents were employed. Lipid extraction from products in which lipids were associated with proteins such as emulsified formulated products or **muscle foods** was cumbersome and time-consuming. Also, inefficient lipid extraction could lead to erroneous analysis of FA composition. If the extraction step could be omitted and FAME could be prepared *in situ* from lipid-containing foods, the simplified procedure would save labour, organic solvent waste and increase sample throughput. Direct FAME preparation without prior lipid extraction was used on microbes and **cereal grains** without comparision to other methods. By heating feedstuffs and faeces in benzene and methanolic HCl, FAME was prepared which had a FA composition comparable to FAME prepared through saponiiication followed by methylation or transesterification of lipid extract. That method, however, required pretreatment of samples for moisture removal in addition to prolonged heating of a reaction mixture (2 hr at 70°C). Moisture at > 2.5 % of the reaction mixture hindered the transesterification reaction. To minimize the interference from water. 2,2-dimethoxypropane was included in the methanolic HCl and improved the transesterification of leaf lipids. However, unreacted reagent was ascribed to spurious peaks on the chromatpgrams. FAME was also prepared by heating **soybean seed meal** in hexane and methanolic sulfuric acid which resulted in < 70 % conversion of the seed oil to methyl esters. This could be due to a relatively short heating time (20 min at 90°C) since a 98 % recovery was obtained with tripalmitin using similar reagents and a longer time of 3 hr at 95°C. Nonetheless, that inference was not persuasive considering the complete methylation of lipids in biological materials exposed to similar reagents at -65°C. By heating lyophilized lipoprotein with methanolic BF_3 (90 min at 110°C), higher FAME yields were obtained than from the transesterification of lipid extract. By heating at 100°C for 60 min various biological specimens in mcthanol-benzene (4:1, v/v) following addition of acetyl chloride. This method, after modification to a milder reaction condition, was used to selectively methylate plasma free FAs.

Compared with acid catalysis, only a few methods had utilized base-catalyzed reagents for direct FAME preparation. This might be partly due to the greater interference of water in base-catalyzed transesterification, because FFAs resulting from lipid hydrolysis were not methylated. Since, methanolic BFs alone or in combination with methanolic NaOH was a popular method to prepare FAME from lipid extract, therefore, *in situ* transesterification was explored through alcoholysis with methanolic NaOH followed by further methylation with methanolic BF_3, which had been successful in preparing FAME directly from ground **peanuts**. The lipid extract was omitted and performed *in situ* transesterification (ISTE) by heating lipid-containing foods at 90°C for 10 min after adding 0.5N NaOH in methanol for methanolysis and continued heating another 10 min for further methylation after adding 14 % BF_3 in methanol. FAME prepared by ISTE showed FA composition virtually identical to FAME prepared after lipid extraction from powder, liquid, phospholipid-rich and tissue products. Due to its simplicity, speed and reduced organic solvent usage, ISTE could be useful to determine overall FA composition of foods.

Interest in milk composition was renewed because of ongoing studies to increase the EFA content, to determine accurately the *tram* content and lately, to quantitate the conjugated octadecadiencs which had been associated with inhibition of **carcinogcnesis** and **tumorigenesis**. Milk and rumen FA compositions were complex. Not only was there a large range in chain length from C_4 to C_{26} (including branch-chain FAs), but also contained many positional and geometric isomers of mono-, di- and tri-unsaturated FAs and many of these FAs were present in very low concentrations. In 1991, 400 FAs were estimated to be present in bovine milk. No single method was available to resolve all these FAs. The availability of long polar capillary columns (50 to 100 mt) for gas-liquid chromatography (GLC) had improved the resolution of many positional and geometric isomers. Prior separations with **argentation chromatography** still showed several regions with overlapping peaks particularly in the mono- and diunsaturated FA region. Difficulties occurred in quantitatively preparing esters from such a great variety of FAs & lipid classes that were present in milk and rumen lipids. Sodium methoxide-catalyzed methylations had been used, but FFAs and N-acyl lipids were not methylated under these conditions. Acid-catalyzed methylations converted all known lipid classes; however, the conjugated dienes were isomerized.

The very short-chain FA methyl esters FAME were difficult to quantitate because the methyl esters were volatile, water-soluble and required correction factors. It was felt for a need of a routine method for the analysis of total milk and rumen FAs, without extensive secondary fractionations. Several acid- and base-catalyzed methylation methods were evaluated for the analyses of milk and rumen lipids. Some of the important criteria were considered - coextraction of artifacts with hexane that might otherwise, interfered with the direct analyses of the hexane extracted by GLC, extent of isomerization of conjugated dienes and methoxy artifact formation as judged by GLC, comparision of total *tram* content determined by GLC and infra-red (IR) spectroscopy. A chromatographic separation was presented using a 100-mt capillary column that resulted in the separation of about 180 peaks from milk lipids. The best compromise for milk FAs was obtained with $NaOCH_3$, followed by HCl or BF3 or diazomethane followed by $NaOCH_3$, being aware that sphingomyelins would be ignored. For rumen samples, the best method suggested was diazomethane followed by $NaOCH_3$.

Bio-Hydrogenation in the artificial-rumen

To be able to stimulate physiological conditions, a full complement of the ruminal microbes was necessary. A naturally compartmented rumen simulation system for the continuous culture of rumen-microbes was used. Ruminal bio-hydrogenation of linoleic acid was monitored in the artificial-rumen (fermenters) with a continuous culture of microbes. Rates of bio-hydrogenation and changes of FAs in culture were measured during steady-state concentration of linoleic acid that was achieved by continuous infusion of known amounts of linoleic acid into the fermenters. A number of *trans* and *cis* isomers were identified using a GLC equipped with an infrared-detector. The infusion of linoleic acid resulted in a substantial increase in the content ot *trans* $C_{18:1}$ and a lesser increase in

cis-$C_{18:1}$. The major *trans* peak consisted of a mixture of n-9 & n-7 isomers. Bio-hydrogenation of infused linoleic acid averaged 77 %. There was evidence of FA-loss, as determined by a decrease in the recovery of linoleic acid after 8 hr of infusion. Addition of $C_{18:2n-6}$ had no major effect on the VFA production by rumen-microbes. The results were similar to those measured *in vivo*, indicating that artificial fermenters were reliable predictors of FA-melabolism *in vivo*.

Chapter 22

Formulation of Premix

A premix is a mixture of vitamins, trace minerals, medicaments, feed supplements and diluents either individually or in a combination. It is a value added solution for feeds with sustainable safety and quality.

The main objective of premixes is to deliver the micro-ingredients in a manner desired by customer. These blends of Micro-ingredients need to be carefully selected, analysed and homogenously manufactured in controlled conditions.

Good quality premixes are manufactured as per following four fundamental principles that determine premix quality and performance :

1. Understanding the chemical and physical attributes in the microingredient to be incorporated.
2. Testing to ensure that all microingredients meet specifications.
3. Controlling the inclusion in fullproof and secure method.
4. Blending together in speciality mixers to achieve a homogenous mix.

Premix Vs Single Ingredients

Whether dry or liquid, standard or customized-premixes can be tailored to meet the needs of every feed manufacturer or finale customer. Choosing a premix formulation over purchasing a selection of single ingredients offers a number of benefits.

Premix manufacturing process comprises:

A. Raw Materials
   1. Selection & Specifications
   2. Purchase
   3. Receipt & Storage
   4. Sampling & Analysis
   5. Processing
B. Formulation
C. Weighing
D. Mixing
E. Packaging
F. Labeling
G. Storage of Finished Premix

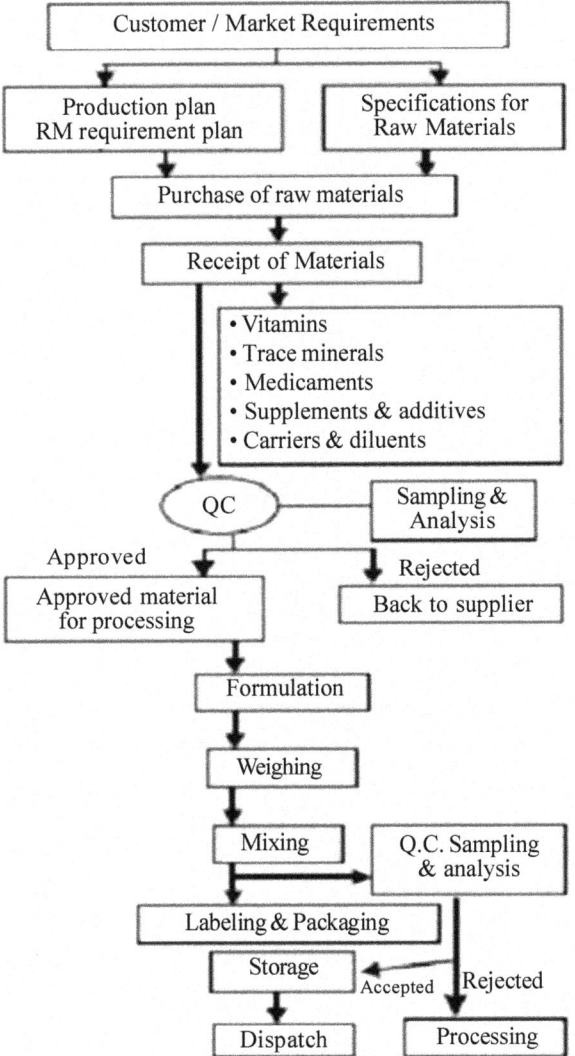

Flow Chart 3 : Flow chart of primix production process

Formulation

This is an important and critical step in manufacturing a premix. Qualified personnel possessing knowledge and expertise regarding micro ingredients and powder technology should formulate a premix.

The formulator has to consider source of ingredients based on their physical, chemical characteristics, bioavailability, their interactions when mixed, handling characteristics, and economic implications on the final product before any final conclusion is arrived at.

Physical Characteristics	Chemical Characteristics
Particle size	Potency
Particle shape	Purity
Particle density	pH
Flowability	Reactivity
Compressibillity	Stability

Physical Characteristics

Particles of uniform size, density and that of spherical shape blend well to form a homogenous mixture. The chance of segregation is thereby minimized.

For example: trace minerals available in the market are invariably found to be coarse in nature whereas the vitamins are normally fine powders. Achieving a homogenous mixing of these two ingredients would be difficult (sand and pebble effect). However, homogenous mixing can be achieved by processing the trace minerals to the desired particle size and improved flowability.

The flow ability of the ingredients plays a vital role while handling the powder i.e. before and after mixing. Poor flow ability results in bridging, caking and product loss in the transfer system. Conversely too, fluid a product may cause flushing.

Chemical Characteristics

Potency of vitamins, trace minerals and medicaments need to be considered whilst formulating high quality premixes. Based on the customer's requirement the formulator has to include the micronutrients considering their analytical value so that desired amount can be delivered when mixed in the feed. No materials should be incorporated in the premix without analysis since under or over addition may have deleterious effect on the overall performance of the birds consuming the feed.

Selection of carrier and its percentage is important for formulating a quality premix. It is generally preferable to leave sufficient space for a carrier in order to minimize any sort of interactions between the active ingredients.

The carrier should serve the functions as depicted below:
- It should neutralize the electrostatic charges present in certain ingredients.
- Chemically inert
- Primarily have the density, particle shape and particle size compatible with other micro ingredients so as to prevent any demixing in the premix.
- Water sequester from other raw materials thereby reducing water activity and improve stability of the premix.

- Impart good flowability. Types of carrier widely used in the formulation of premix :
A. Organic carriers
B. Inorganic carriers

Organic Carriers	Inorganic Carriers
Wheat middling	Calcium carbonate
Rice hulls	Cicalcium phosphate
Corn cobb, ground	Monocalcium phosphate
Soya bean meal	Meolite
Lactose	Fine dried salt

Better premixes can often be prepared by employing a blend of predetermined ratio of several diluents rather than with just one. The organic carrier absorbs moisture while inorganic carrier contributes towards density of premix.

The formulator has to consider all the above-mentioned parameters whilst preparing the batch control or manufacturing record. The batch manufacturing record serves as a link between the formulator and actual production. While preparing the batch sheet the formulator has to give importance for the following details:

- Nutrient requirements
- Selection of ingredients
- Potency of ingredient
- Process loss
- Level of free flowing agents
- Level of antioxidant
- Percentage of carrier
- Packing & packaging material
- Inventory of materials

The manufacturing of a premix should follow the batch control sheet under the supervision of trained personnel. The batch sheet should comprise following details:

- Name of the premix
- Code of premix
- Production date
- Batch no. of premix

Formulation of Premix

- Batch size
- List of ingredients to be mixed
- Batch no. of ingredients to be mixed
- Mixing order of ingredients
- Actual quantity of ingredients to be taken
- Mixer name and mixing time
- Instructions regarding packing and mixing
- Provision for signatures

All the above-mentioned details aid in keeping a track of the premix which may be traced in future with respect to customer complaints or product recall. Thus it serves as a control copy.

Some premix feeds used in cattle

1. *Vitamin Premix As Feed Additive Cattle*

Feedex : Feedex is specifically developed to provide optimum nutrition for Ruminants during their entire productive life through feeds. They include fortification levels that meet the vitamin needs of ruminants for optimum health and productivity in real time situation.

Composition : Each 250 gmContains:Vitamin A- 12500000 I.U., Vitamin D3 -2500000 I.U., Vitamin E -50000 I.U., Vitamin B12 -25000 mcg, Vitamin K -1000 I.U., Niacin- 12000 mg, Biotin- 10000 mcg

Dosage : 250 gm per ton of feed

2. *Cattle liquid vitamin and mineral supplementation*

Covit: Fat soluble vitamins & Trace minerals play a significant role in better conception rate and productivity of dairy animals and for better growth and optimum health in the young animals. Hence, it is recommended to supplement daily rations of dairy animals

Composition : Combination of Vitamin A, D3, E, Biotin, Zinc, Cobalt, Selenium, D.L. Methionine & L-Lysine.

Dosage: Calves: 5 ml per day per Animal

Large Animal: 10 ml per day per Animal

3. *Chelated Minerals and Vitamin Supplementation*

Bovimax: Delivers specific nutrients to precise targets such as the rumen, the liver, the immune system, reproductive organs & hoof horn. The low productivity in animals is mainly due to nutritional factors out of which more than 40% could be attributed to the mineral imbalances.

Composition: Combination of essential Chelated Trace Minerals along with Macro Minerals, Vitamins, By Pass Fat & By Pass Protein.

Dosage: 50 gm per day per animal or 1 kg per 100 kg of feed

4. *Organic Trace Mineral Supplementation*

Protomin BS: The modern genetic breeds have increased productivity levels, improving growth speed, profits and animal quality. As a result, nutritional requirements have been increasing too. Animals are frequently subjected to dietary deficiencies of trace elements like copper, cobalt, manganese, and iron.

Composition: Each 1 kg Contains:

Copper-4.2 gm, Cobalt-200 mg, Iron-6.0 gm, Zinc-9.6 gm, Magnesium-50.0 gm, Manganese-1.5 gm, Iodine-1.0 gm, Methionine-10.0 gm, Lysine-10.0 gm, Yeast culture as required with fortified base.

Chapter 23

Mechanic's of Feed Mixing

This procedure allows us to mix two feed stuffs with different nutrient concentrations and come up with a mixture of the desired total concentration. For this square to work, the desired diet nutrient concentration must be between the nutrient concentrations of the two feed stuffs as well as in the same unit. The procedure can be used for Crude Protein, Energy, Minerals and so on and so forth. Also, in place of percentage, calories, parts per million / billion / trillion and other units of measurement can be used.

Double Pearson Square Method

Sometimes, we might want to have the exact amounts of two major nutrients such as - Crude Protein and Energy.

For example, suppose we want a final mixture with 12 % Crude Protein (CP) and 74 % Total Digestible Nutrient (T.D.N.). We have :

1. Corn	with 8.8 % CP	and 81 % TDN
2. Cotton Seed Meal (CSM)	with 40.9 % CP	and 68.6 % TDN
3. Oat hay	with 8.1 % CP	and 53.8% TDN

For this, we must have a minimum of three feed stuffs

First, we go through two squares and get a mixture exact for each nutrient. In this example, we shall do CP first. We must have one mixture with 12 % CP and greater than 74 % TDN; and another mixture with 12 % CP and less than 74 % TDN. We proceed as shown :

Mixture 1   12 % CP,   > 74 % TDN

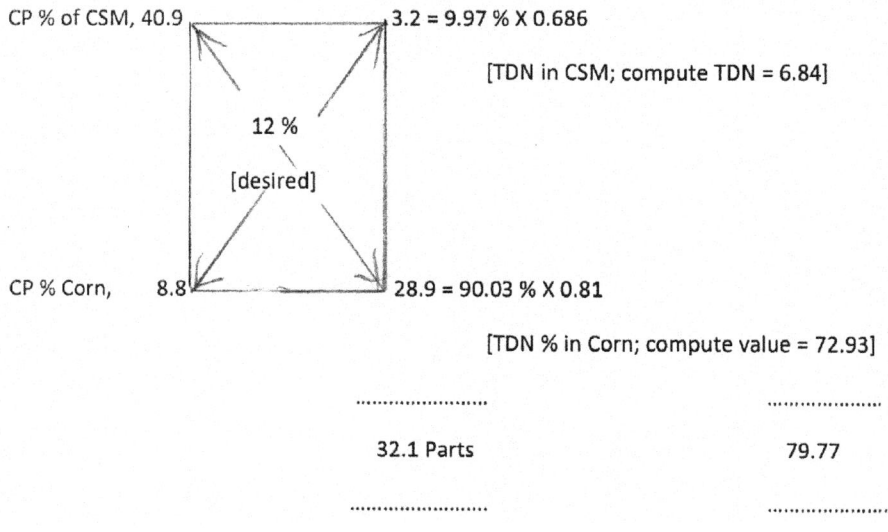

Mixture 2   12 % CP,   < 74 % TDN

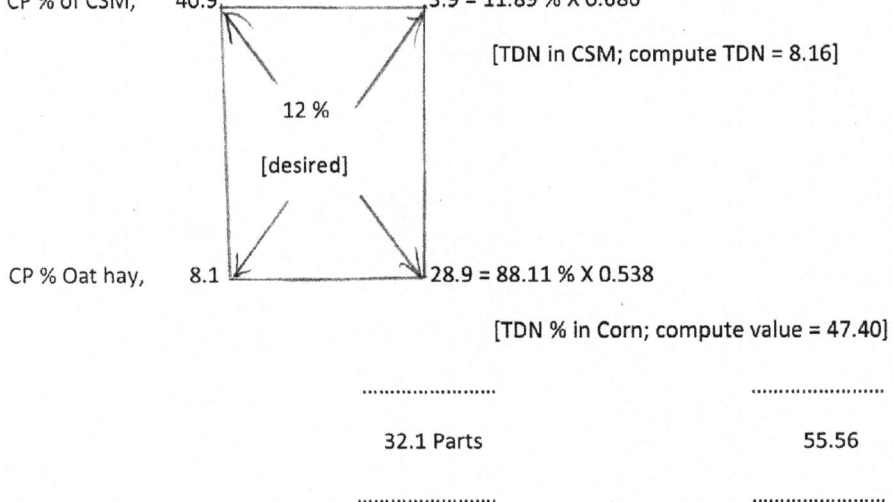

Then solve for TDN in the third square :

Mixture 3   12 % CP and   74 % TDN

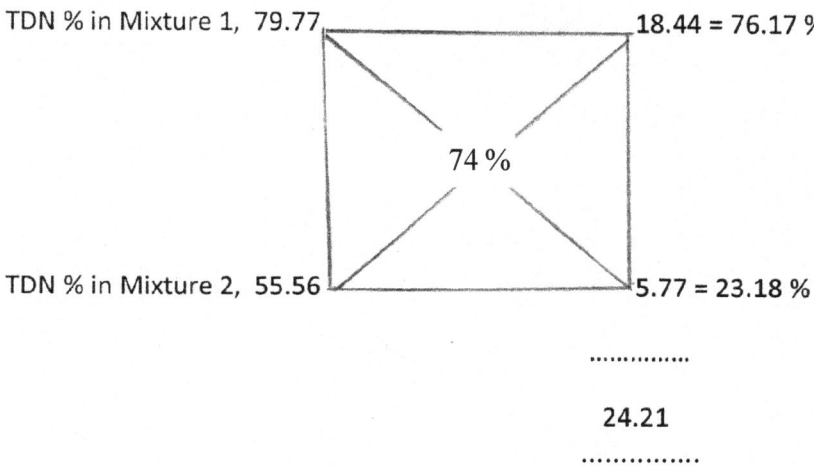

TDN % in Mixture 1, 79.77   18.44 = 76.17 %

74 %

TDN % in Mixture 2, 55.56   5.77 = 23.18 %

                                           ....
                                           24.21
                                           ....

Now, ingredient composition can be calculated -

CSM % in Mixture 1,   9.97 X 0.762

                 [76.17 % of Mixture 1 in Mixture 3] = 7.594

CSM % in Mixture 2,   11.89 X 0.238

                 [23.83 % of Mixture 2 in Mixture 3] = 2.833

                                             ....

CSM in Mixture 1 and Mixture 2   = 10.427

                                                   ≈ 10.43

                                                        (rounded off)

Corn % in Mixture **1 and Oat** % **in Mixture 2**

Corn % in Mixture 1, 90.03 X 0.762

[76.17 % of Mixture 1 and Mixture 3] = 68.57

Oat % in Mixture 2, 88.83 % X 0.238

[23.83 % of Mixture 2 in Mixture 3] = 21.00

Now, check CP [using composition table]

= 10.42 X 0.409 + 68.57 X 0.088 + 21 X 0.08

= 4.27 + 6.03 + 1.70

= 11.98

= **12.00**

Now, check CP [using composition table]

= 10.427 X 0.686 + 68.57 X 0.81 + 21 X 0.538

= 7.16 + 55.54+11.30

= **74.00**

[If more nutrients are there, then computer would be required].

Chapter 24

Automated Mill

A **mill** is a device that breaks solid materials into smaller pieces by grinding, crushing, or cutting. Such communition is an important unit operation in many processes. There are many different types of mills and many types of materials processed in them. Historically, mills were powered by hand (e.g., via hand cranks) working animals (horsemill), wind (wind mill) or water (watermill). Today they are usually powered by electricity and are controlled by computer (automatic mills).

The grinding of solid matters occurs under exposure of mechanical forces that trench the structure by overcoming of the interior bonding forces. After the grinding, the state of the solid is changed: the grain size, the grain size disposition and the grain shape.

Milling also refers to the process of breaking down, separating, sizing, or classifying aggregate material. For instance rock crushing or grinding to produce uniform aggregate size for construction purposes, or separation of rock, soil or aggregate material for the purposes of structural fill or land reclamation activities. Aggregate milling processes are also used to remove or separate contamination or moisture from aggregate or soil and to produce "dry fills" prior to transport or structural filling.

Grinding may serve the following purposes in engineering:
- Increase of the surface area of a solid
- Manufacturing of a solid with a desired grain size
- Pulping of resources

Many feed companies focussed on automation of batching and pelleting process. In current climate of rising feed ingredient costs, risking labour cost, rising energy costs, there is opportunity for significant economic benefits through complete process automation. To relies the full benefits of automation the production process should be expanded to include the order processing and production planning, raw material receiving, raw material storage and transfer for blending grinding, interface with formulation system for real time production adjustment, routing to finished products silos and packing, truck loading (bulk and bags) delivery and logistic.

As well as the benefits of complete traceability and total feed safety complete automation can provide following:

Weekly daily hourly updates stock inventories and tolerance.

Interface with SAP/formulation and other management information system to provide multiple reporting options.

Effective management and security of all trucks and personnel entering/leaving the site.

More effective response to QA and impact on the formulation and production costs.

Reduction in labours costs, power cost and losses associated with stock inventory variance.

The feed mill of the future will not survive based on the current best practice. Feed mill automation can provide significant advantage if viewed as an holistic management tool. Every part of the process needs to be accountable in real time. Ability to interact with other management system will expand the opportunities associated with purchasing/formulating and logistics.

Grinding machines

In materials processing a **grinder** is a machine for producing fine particle size reduction through attrition and compressive force at the grain size level and crusher for mechanisms producing larger particles. In general, grinding processes require a relatively large amount of energy; for this reason, an experimental method to measure the energy used locally during milling with different machines was recently proposed.

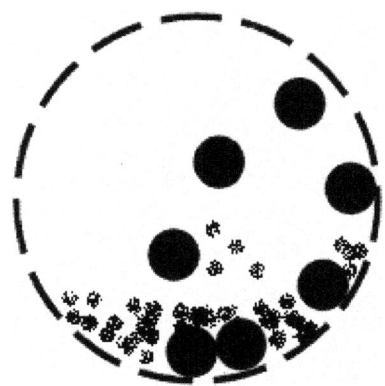

Operation of a ball mill

Ball mill A typical type of fine grinder is the ball mill. A slightly inclined or horizontal rotating cylinder is partially filled with balls, usually stone or metal which grind material to the necessary fineness by friction and impact with the tumbling balls. Ball mills normally operate with an approximate ball charge of 30%. Ball mills are characterized by their smaller (comparatively) diameter and longer length, and often have a length 1.5 to 2.5 times the diameter. The feed is at one end of the cylinder and the discharge is at the other. Ball mills are commonly used in the manufacture of Portland cement and finer grinding stages of mineral processing. Industrial ball mills can be as large as 8.5 m (28 ft) in diameter with a 22 MW motor drawing approximately 0.0011% of the total world's power. However, small versions of ball mills can be found in laboratories where they are used for grinding sample material for quality assurance.

Rod mill A rotating drum causes friction and attrition between steel rods and ore particles. But the term 'rod mill' is also used as a synonym for a slitting mill which makes rods of iron or other metal. Rod mills are less common than ball mills for grinding minerals. The rods used in the mill, usually a high-carbon steel, can vary in both the length and the diameter. However, the smaller the rods, the larger is the total surface area and hence, the greater the grinding efficiency.

Autogenous mills

Autogenous or autogenic mills are so-called due to the self-grinding of the ore: a rotating drum throws larger rocks of ore in a cascading motion which causes impact breakage of larger rocks and compressive grinding of finer particles. It is similar in operation to a SAG mill as described below but does not use steel balls in the mill. Also known as ROM or "Run Of Mine" grinding.

SAG mills

SAG is an acronym for Semi-Autogenous Grinding. SAG mills are autogenous mills but use grinding balls like a ball mill. A SAG mill is usually a primary or first stage grinder. SAG mills use a ball charge of 8 to 21%. The largest SAG mill is 42' (12.8m) in diameter, powered by a 28 MW (38,000 HP) motor. A SAG mill with a 44' (13.4m) diameter and a power of 35 MW (47,000 HP) has been designed.

Attrition between grinding balls and ore particles causes grinding of finer particles. SAG mills are characterized by their large diameter and short length as compared to ball mills. The inside of the mill is lined with lifting plates to lift the material inside the mill, where it then falls off the plates onto the rest of the ore charge. SAG mills are primarily used at gold, copper and platinum mines with applications also in the lead, zinc, silver, alumina and nickel industries.

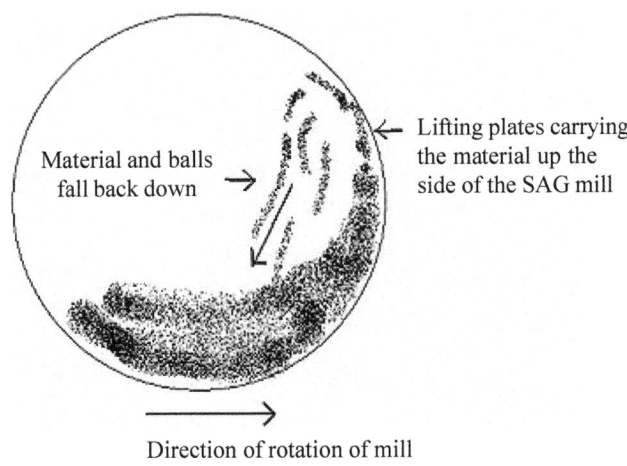

Principle of SAG Mill operation

Pebble mill

A rotating drum causes friction and attrition between rocks pebbles and ore particles. May be used where product contamination by iron from steel balls must be avoided. Quartz or silica is commonly used because it is inexpensive to obtain.

High pressure grinding rolls

A high pressure grinding roll, often referred to as roller press consists out of two rollers with the same dimensions, which are rotating against each other with the same circumferential speed. The special feeding of bulk material through a hopper leads to a material bed between the two rollers. The bearing units of one roller can move linearly and are pressed against the material bed by springs or hydraulic cylinders. The pressures in the material bed are greater than 50 MPa (7,000 PSI). In general they achieve 100 to 300 MPa. By this the material bed is compacted to a solid volume portion of more than 80%.The roller press has a certain similarity to roller crushers and roller presses for the compacting of powders, but purpose, construction and operation mode are different.Extreme pressure causes the particles inside of the compacted material bed to fracture into finer particles and also causes microfracturing at the grain size level. Compared to ball mills HPGRs achieve a 30 to 50% lower specific energy consumption, although they are not as common as ball mills since they are a newer technology. A similar type of intermediate crusher is the edge runner, which consists of a circular pan with two or more heavy weels known as mullers rotating within it; material to be crushed is shoved underneath the wheels using attached blades.

Buhrstone mill

Table top hammer millanother type of fine grinder commonly used is the buharstone mills which is similar to old-fashioned flour mills.

Vertical shaft impactor mill (VSI mill)

A VSI mill throws rock or ore particles against a wear plate by slinging them from a spinning center that rotates on a vertical shaft. This type of mill uses the same principle as VSI crusher.

Tower mill Tower mills, often called vertical mills, stirred mills or regrind mills, are a more efficient means of grinding material at smaller particle sizes, and can be used after ball mills in a grinding process. Like ball mills, grinding (steel) balls or pebbles are often added to stirred mills to help grind ore, however these mills contain a large screw mounted vertically to lift and grind material. In tower mills, there is no cascading action as in standard grinding mills. Stirred mills are also common for mixing quicklime (CaO) into lime slurry. There are several advantages to the tower mill: low noise, efficient energy usage, and low operating costs.

STEPS

Raw Ingredient- Receiving Feed mills typically receive incoming ingredients by both rail and truck (including hopper bottom, bulk solids, and liquids trailers). Typically major (such as grain and soybean meal) and minor ingredients (such as lime, brewer's grains, wheat midds, etc.) will be received via these systems. Micro-ingredients, such as minerals, are commonly delivered via bulk truck and then pneumatically conveyed to the appropriate storage bins. This type of system requires blowers, delivery lines, receivers, filters, and airlocks; typically one system for each ingredient to be received.

Grinding : Prior to utilization in feed formulations, whole grain must be ground to reduce particle size. Grinding systems are generally located directly under whole grain storage bins, in a separate room within the mill facility (Figure 1), or in a separate grinding building adjacent to the mill structure. Roller mills have been gaining in popularity over the last several years, primarily because of their ability to produce coarse, uniform particle sizes, with reduced noise levels, and with reduced power consumption.

Batching : In order to produce particular feed mixtures, appropriate quantities of specific ingredients must be transferred out of storage and transported to the mixer. This is the function of the batching system. For all major and minor ingredients, the equipment used to accomplish this includes screw feeders (e.g., screw conveyors), which provide excellent proportioning control, and are thus the conveyor of choice for this operation, and scale hoppers, which are hoppers mounted on load cells above the mixer. These hoppers range in size from one ton up to 5 tons, and must be designed with slopes greater than 60 degree C, to prevent ingredient build-up.

Mixing : To produce specified feed mixtures, most modern feed mills utilize horizontal batch ribbon mixers, which have bottom gates that dump directly into a conveyor (typically a paddle drag) that transfers the mixed feed (e.g., mash) to a bucket elevator, where it is elevated and distributed to appropriate storage bins. Mash resides in storage until needed for pelleting, bagging, or direct bulk loadout. Ribbon mixers vary in size, but can be constructed as large as 700 ft3 in capacity.

Pelleting : Pelleting is a process intended to densify feed ingredients, which will improve storage, handling, and shipping behavior, and to improve the feed nutritionally by increasing the palatability and feed efficiency in the livestock. Typically mixed feed (e.g., mash) is transported from the mash storage bins to a preconditioner, where it is mixed with steam so that it is more amenable to the pelleting process. Residence time in a conditioner of 20 sec is recommended, but various plants often use longer times. After conditioning the feed particles, they are then introduced into the pellet mill, where a rotating roller forces the ingredients through circular die openings, which typically have diameters smaller than ¾ in. Modern pellet mills can have die diameters up to 42 in, with effective pelleting surfaces of 1600 in2, can produce pelleted feed at a rate of up to 50 ton/h, and can consume up to 800 hp.

Cooling : After processing, the pellets are then cooled (horizontal or counterflow coolers are generally used), so that pellet temperature is reduced to ambient (in order to avoid spoilage problems), screened to removed fines and broken pellets, and then conveyed to storage, after which they will either be bagged or loaded out in bulk.

Crumbling : Cooled pellets may be ground on corrugated rolls and the resulting product sifted into various sizes of granules or crumbles

Packaging : Feed packaging machine is used to complete the feed packaging process in the large and medium feed mill .Feed bagging machine includes the filling, weighting, delivering and sealing process. Bagged feed pellets is easy to store and transport. More important it can prevent feed pellets from damp, corrosion and oxidation.

Chapter 25

Problems and Quarantine Measures in Feed Mills

Introduction

First feed mill was established in 1875 A.D. in the state of Illinois, U.S.A. for calf meal production.

First feed mill in India was established in Ludhiana, Punjab in 1969 A.D.

Processing of Ingredients in Mill

Flow chart of processing:

Receiving
↓
Grinding
↓
Mixing
↓
Processing
↓
Packaging → Bulk Head Out
↓
Warehouse

Receiving

There are certain hazards which should be checked during the receiving of the ingredients which would come
- Under hazard assessment.

Bulk Ingredient Receiving

1. BIOLOGICAL- fungal growth
   - Pests
   - Rodents
2. PHYSICAL - ferrous meatal
   - Non ferrous metal
   - Glass
   - Stones
3. CHEMICAL - aflatoxin
   - Vomitoxin
   - Fumanisin
4. OTHER- incorrect product received
   - Cross-contamination from previous loads.

Monitoring/Inspection

1. Documentation
2. Visual inspection of bulk
1. TRUCK bagged receiving hand add BULK drugs
2. OPERATOR recording QA supervisor (RECORDS)
3. DAILY & ANNUAL AUDIT daily daily + monthy + annual audit

HACCP

1. Hazard analysis
2. Control points
3. Critical limits
4. Monitoring
5. Verification procedure
6. Recording

Control Measure & Facilities

1. There must be covered area for the processing of the ingredients in the mill.
2. Recording & documentation should be proper.
3. Use of insecticides to control insects- spray of melathione 50%, 10 ml in 1 liter water on empty gunny bags.
4. Fumigation using ethylene dibromide & ecofume.
5. Rodenticides : anti coagulant – warfarin. & Zn sulfate.

Chapter 26

Use of Computer on Feed Formulation

Introduction
- Objective of animal diet formulations to provide a palatable ration at minimum cost to meet nutritional and energy requirements of the animal.
- To achieve this objective, it is important to have knowledge about the requirements of specific nutrient ingredients and the nutrient composition of feeds, which are used to formulate the animal diet.
- Diet formulation is an important aspect to meet production and financial goals in the most economical way.
- A diet is called balanced if it provides energy to meet lactation, production and specific level of health requirement.
- Economic as well as nutritional aspects should be considered while optimising nutrient ingredients.
- These three factors are so intimately related to each other that cannot be separated during the process of feed formulation.

Preliminary Stages
- The first step in diet formulation is to define the objective of diet formulation. Depending on the objective of diet formulation (such as reproduction, lactation, live-stock etc.), requirements for nutrient ingredients are established
- This step includes individual units and overall requirement for diet ingredients. After defining the objective of study and diet formulation, requirements of nutrient intake are defined to achieve that objective
- While defining the requirement, social environment, internal, external and economical conditions should be taken into consideration. Nutrient requirements can be established by the empirical method and factorial method.
- The empirical method is based on experimental studies whereas the factorial method identifies the various functions within the animal that defines the needs of nutrient ingredients.

Ingredient Selection and Diet Formulation

- Once requirements for nutrient ingredients are established, the ingredients can be selected and nutrient contents calculated.
- After identifying the nutrient ingredients, diet is formulated by using existing methods and different mathematical techniques. There are different methods to formulate animal diet.
- Diet formulation includes balance mixture of ingredients which are economically sustainable and provides nutrient and energy requirements of a given species for a given response. Different kind of conventional methods to formulate the diets include:
    - Trial-and-error method
    - Two by two matrix method
    - Square method
    - Simultaneous equation method
    - Least cost formulation
    - Linear programming method
- Initially, feed manufacturers for animal feed formulation used the trial and error method but this included tedious hand calculations.

Diet Analysis and Evaluation

- After formulation, the diet is evaluated to check the efficiency of diet. Chemical analysis is done to check whether the diet is mixed correctly or not. These five steps of diet formulation .By employing the correct formulation skills and techniques, animal performance can be improved. These are two important aspects, which make a huge impact on the overall profitability. Whether diet is formulated for feed milers or integrators, maximisation of animal production is important.By the end of the 1960s, wide spread use of linear programming had been started for animal diet formulation. To take into account the complexity and nutrient variability, different kinds of mathematical programming came into the picture with the objective of least cost rationing. To achieve this, different kinds of mathematical programming have been used. For example, linear programming, non-linear programming, stochastic programming sensitivity analysis, parametric cost and nutrient ranging, optimum-density formulation, multi-blending, and risk analysis.Chance constrained programming is used to formulate commercial feeds for animals. The linear programming model can be solved for a complicated set of nutrient requirements to give a relatively well-balanced ration. Alteration in the diet formulation can change undefined nutrient or dietary components, such as fatty acids, phytoestrogens, phytosterols, nitrosamines and methyl mercury, potentially affecting research outcomes.

Computer-aided Feed Formulation

- A study was conducted for animal feed formulation based on internet remote and interaction by Xiong Benhai, Luo Qing-yao and Pang Zhihong in 2002. This program is based on linear programming, with SQL Server 2000 database and ASP Web-page language Windows 2000 Advanced Server. The most important feature of this system is that it has set up one whole calculating platform to design all kinds formulas based on web technique, which can share information of feed science and animal nutrition to help directly designing feed formulas. A computer program called APOLLO was developed by A. Ahmadi, J.R. Dunbar and H.A. Johnson for formulation and analysis of ration for swine. This program runs on IBM PC compatible computers with 512K of memory. After feeding the input nutrient ingredients,

- This program formulates the ration using the linear programming primal dual algorithm. This algorithm is efficient in time and space because it does not require additional columns and rows for artificial variables. The output consists of five parts :cost and performance, ration composition, price ranges, nutrient analysis of the ration and nutrient analysis of feeds in the ration which, in turn, consists of eight parts.

Practical and Economic Implications

- In the 1980s, the first computer program was presented for animal diet formulation. Since then, a number of computer programs have been developed for the purpose of animal diet formulation which discusses specific feed formulation techniques in terms of their practical applications and economic implications. The use of computer programming lessened the time and effort required to provide affordable feed formulations for the feed industry. A wide variety of computer programs are available for ration formulation. Moreover, **computer programming for animal diet formulation is easy, convenient and saves time**. A number of nutrient ingredients and constraints can be added to a diet in easier manner. It is also possible to check the impact of different nutrient ingredients on animal production without actually applying it with the help of a computer program.

The Language of Programming

- To initiate the process of computer programming for animal diet formulation, a mathematical model is formulated which should be nutritionally adequate at lowest cost. When formulating this mathematical model, availability of feedstuffs, physical palatability, toxicological properties of feed logistics of obtaining feed ingredients and storage limit should be considered. After creating the mathematical model, computer programming is to be chosen for this purpose. A number of programming languages have been used for this purpose as C, C++, Java and MATLAB.

Using C for Feed Formulation

- One of the most basic and important programming languages is referred as 'C'. Dennis Ritchie developed this programming language at Bell Laboratories in 1972. Many of its principles and ideas were based on the earlier language B and B's earlier ancestor BCPL and CPL. The main features of this language are its flexibility that provides fast program execution and the lack of constraints it imposes on the programmer. It allows low level access to information and commands while still retaining the portability and syntax of a high level language. It is useful for both systems programming and general purpose programs. Due to this quality of C language, the Unix operating system, which was originally written in assembly language, was almost immediately rewritten in C. C includes bit-wise operators along with powerful pointer manipulation capabilities and modularity Is another important feature of this language. Sections of code can be stored in libraries for re-use in future programs. This language is very useful for animal diet formulation because of its easily applicable features. A programming technique is developed for animal diet formulation using non-linear programming and C language with the objective of maximum animal weight gain. The technique presented formulates and solve a non-linear program with optimum use of nutrient ingredients. It explores the use of mathematical and computerised programming in the field of animal nutrition and can be investigated in future for more variables.

The Advantages of Matlab

- MATLAB is another tool for matrix manipulations, and interfacing with programs written in other languages, including C and Java. It is a high-level language for numerical computation, visualization, and application development. Animal feed is formalated using MATLAB with the objective of maximum animal weight gain. In the first step, this technique involves formulation of objective function using non-linear programming. MATLAB is used as a tool for this purpose. In the second step, the solution of formulation is given and is compared to existing techniques. Use of non-linear programming overcomes the drawback of linear approximation of objective function

- In the present era of technology, it is convenient, time and money saving to take benefits of computer programming for this purpose. Using this technology animal diet formulation can be simulated and experiments can be done with the help of computer programs, without hampering the existing system of feeding to the animal and could reach to better results.

Chapter 27

Codex Alimentarius

The Codex alimentarius is a collection of standards, codes of practice, guidelines and other recommendations relative to food.

It is derived from **latin word** which means **Food Code**.

Codex alimentarius is about safe, good food for everyone - everywhere.

International food trade has existed for thousands of years but until not too long ago food was mainly produced, sold and consumed locally. Over the last century the amount of food traded internationally has grown exponentially, and a quantity and variety of food never before possible travels the globe today.

The CODEX ALIMENTARIUS international food standards, guidelines and codes of practice contribute to the safety, quality and fairness of this international food trade. Consumers can trust the safety and quality of the food products they buy and importers can trust that the food they ordered will be in accordance with their specifications.

Public concerns about food safety issues are often placing Codex at the centre of global debates. Biotechnology, pesticides, food additives and contaminants are some of the issues discussed in Codex meetings. Codex standards are based on the best available science assisted by independent international risk assessment bodies or ad-hoc consultations organized by FAO and WHO.

While being recommendations for voluntary application by members, Codex standards serve in many cases as a basis for national legislation.

The reference made to Codex food safety standards in the World Trade Organization's Agreement on Sanitary and Phytosanitary measures (SPS Agreement) means that Codex has far reaching implications for resolving trade disputes. WTO members that wish to apply stricter food safety measures than those set by Codex may be required to justify these measures scientifically.

Codex members cover 99% of the world's population. More and more developing countries are taking an active part in the Codex process - in many cases assisted by the Codex Trust Fund, which strives to finance - and train - participants from such countries to enable efficient participation. Being an active member of Codex helps countries to compete in sophisticated world markets - and to improve food safety for their own population. At the same time exporters know what importers demand, and importers are protected from substandard shipments.

International governmental and non-governmental organizations can become accredited Codex observers to provide expert information, advice and assistance to the Commission.

Since its beginnings in 1963, the Codex system has evolved in an open, transparent and inclusive way to meet emerging challenges. International food trade is a 200 billion dollar a year industry, with billions of tonnes of food produced, marketed and transported.

There is a lot at stake for protecting consumers' health and ensuring fair practices in the food trade.

All information on Codex is public and free. For any questions please contact the Codex Secretariat.

Codex Alimentarius Commission

The Codex alimentarius Commission was born of necessity. its carefully crafted statutes and rules of Procedure ensure that it pursues its clearly defined objectives in a disciplined, dispassionate and scientific way.

The Codex Alimentarius Commission was established by the Food and Agriculture Organization (FAO) and the World Health Organization (WHO) to implement their joint food standards programme and held its first session in 1963. The legal basis for the Commission is contained in the ten articles that form the Statutes of the Codex Alimentarius Commission.

The Codex Alimentarius Commission shall be responsible for making proposals to, and shall be consulted by, the Directors-General of the Food and Agriculture Organization (FAO) and the World Health Organization (WHO) on all matters pertaining to the implementation of the Joint FAO/WHO Food Standards Programme, the purpose of which is:

a) Protecting the health of consumers and ensuring fair practices in the food trade;

b) Promoting coordination of all food standards work undertaken by international governmental and non-governmental organizations;

c) Determining priorities and initiating and guiding the preparation of draft standards through and with the aid of appropriate organizations;

d) Finalizing standards elaborated under (c) above and publishing them in a Codex Alimentarius either as regional or worldwide standards, together with international standards already finalized by other bodies under (b) above, wherever this is practicable;

e) Amending published standards, as appropriate, in the light of developments. From their beginnings, Fao and WHo have promoted the improvement of quality and safety standards applied to food. the highest priority of the Codex alimentarius Commission is to protect the health of consumers.

Codex Members and Observers

Currently the Codex Alimentarius Commission has:

188 Codex Members - 187 Member Countries and 1 Member Organization [European Union (EU)] 219 Codex Observers - 56 IGOs, 147 NGOs, 16 UN.

Members

Membership of the Commission is open to all Member Nations and Associate Members of FAO and WHO which are interested in international food standards. Regional economic integration organizations that are members of either FAO or WHO can also become members and special rules apply. To apply for membership please click here.

Observer nations

Any Member Nation or Associate Member of FAO or WHO which is not a Member of the Commission, may, upon request, attend sessions of the Commission and of its subsidiary bodies and ad hoc meetings as observers. Nations which, while not Member Nations or Associate Members of FAO or WHO, are members of the United Nations, may be invited on their request to attend meetings of the Commission as observers. To request an invitation interested Nations should write to the Codex Secretariat at least one month before the session.

In 2013, Codex celebrated its 50th anniversary-50 years of setting standards to protect consumer health and ensure fair practices in the food trade. For over 50 years thousands of experts from all over the world have dedicated themselves to building and refining the Codex system of international food standards bringing us closer to a world where food is safe, of good quality and available-in every home.

The best traditions of the Food and Agriculture Organization of the United Nations (FAO) and the World Health Organization (WHO) have encouraged food-related scientific and technological research as well as discussion. In doing so, they have lifted the world community's awareness of food safety and related issues to unprecedented heights. The Codex Alimentarius Commission, established by the two Organizations in the 1960s, has become the single most important international reference point for developments associated with food standards.

UN General Assembly stated that where possible Governments should adopt Codex Alimentarius Standards.

FAO/WHO International Conference on Nutrition recognized that food regulations should take into account the recommended international standards of the Codex Alimentarius Commission.

FAO World Food Summit committed to apply measures, in conformity with the Agreement on the Application of Sanitary and Phytosanitary Measures and other relevant international agreements, that ensure the quality and safety of food supply.

FAO/WHO Conference on Food standards recognized the importance of providing evaluations based on sound science and risk assessment principles

Agreement on the Application of Sanitary and Phytosanitary Measures and Agreement on Technical Barriers to Trade formally recognized International standards, guidelines and recommendations, including the Codex Alimentarius, as reference points for facilitating international trade and resolving trade disputes in international law.

53th World Health Assembly recognized the importance of the standards, guidelines and other recommendations of the Codex Alimentarius Commission for protecting the health of consumers and assuring fair trading practices.

The Codex Score Card

The codex Alimentarius Commission has 191 Commodity Standards, 73 Guidelines, 51 Codes of Practice, 17 Maximum levels for contaminants in food, 301 Food additives, 4347 Maximum residue limits for pesticide residues, 610 MRLs for residues of Veterinary drugs in foods.

Codex standards and related texts are voluntary in nature. They need to be translated into national legislation or regulations in order to be enforceable. Codex standards can be general or specific. General Standards, Guidelines and Codes of Practice are applied transversely. These texts deal with hygienic practice, labelling, additives, inspection & certification, nutrition and residues of veterinary drugs and pesticides. Codex commodity standards refer to a specific product although increasingly Codex now develops standards for food groups i.e. one general standard for fruit juices and nectars as opposed to one per fruit.

Codex methods of analysis and sampling, including those for contaminants and residues of pesticides and veterinary drugs in foods, are also considered Codex standards.

Codex guidelines fall into two categories: principles that set out policy in certain key areas; and guidelines for the interpretation of these principles or for the interpretation of the provisions of the Codex general standards.

In the cases of food additives, contaminants, food hygiene and meat hygiene, the basic principles governing the regulation of these matters are built into the relevant standards and codes of practice.

An example of a Codex guideline would be Guidelines for the Design and Implementation of National Regulatory Food Safety Assurance Programmes Associated with the Use of Veterinary Drugs in Food Producing Animals.

Codex codes of practice - including codes of hygienic practice – define the production, processing, manufacturing, transport and storage practices for individual foods or groups of foods that are considered essential to ensure the safety and suitability of food for consumption. For example, for food hygiene, the basic text is the Codex General Principles of Food Hygiene, which introduces the use of the Hazard Analysis and Critical Control Point (HACCP) food safety management system. Another example of a code of practice is the Code of Practice for the Reduction of Acrylamide in Foods

General standards deal primarily with food safety, consumer information and trade requirements. Commodity standards have a common format stating what the commodity is, how it is made and what it may contain.

According to Fao trade statistics, the value of trade in food exceeded Us$ 1.12 trillion in 2013 and is increasing.

"The publication of the Codex Alimentarius is intended to guide and promote the elaboration and establishment of definitions and requirements for foods to assist in their harmonization and in doing so to facilitate international trade."

FAO and WHO complement the Commission's activities significantly in a number of practical ways. FAO and WHO not only support but also help developing countries to apply Codex standards, to strengthen their national food control systems and take advantage of international food trade opportunities.

Chapter 28

Biohydrogenation

Historical Aspect

The primitive man during his long history as a hunter and food gatherer, used ruminants as food till about 6000 B.C. Later, he developed the arts of aerable - agriculture and animal husbandry. The ruminants played a major role as sources of both food and mechanical work. In turn, the new techniques of food production greatly increased the amount of food available and enabled the establishment of settled communities. The radical nature of these developments was clearly shown by the fact that within a couple of millennia, man had evolved from primitive to urbanized, civilized communities. Throughout the historical epochs, animal food - meat, milk and milk products continued to form an important fraction of the diet in most of the civilized societies. The favoured nature of these foods was well shown in the observation that, with increasing affluence, human - beings tended to increase the fraction of the diet provided by animal foods, especially from ruminants.

Since middle of twentieth century, evidences had been accumulating to indicate that the high intake of saturated fats from meat and 'dairy products might play a role in the etiology of atherosclerosis. This concern had provided a stimulus to produce husbandry techniques leading to the modification of the composition of ruminant fats as well as possibility of protecting dietary poly - unsaturated fatty acids (PUFA) from ruminal biohydrogenation in 1951. Scientists all the world round, started studying ruminant fats and ruminal lipid metabolism in this perspective. Different research groups developed various techniques of protecting dietary - PUFA, so as to make them available in the meat, milk and its products, but lacked the availability of sensitive techniques for confirmation. With the discovery of Gas Chromatoaraphy (GC) in 1954, a new beginning of resolution and detection of PUFA started with gradual precision. Later on, the GC was further equipped with mass - spectroscopy and subsequently with infra - red detector. The scientists were very much successful in protecting the dietary essential fatty acids (E.F.A.s) or even by - passing them from biohydrogenation *in vitro*.

Ruminant Fats

The adepocytes were characterized by a high content of stearic acid, isomers of C-18 Unsaturated fatty acids, branched chain fatty acids and acids with odd number of carbon atoms, which due to metabolic changes in the rumen. Following are some findings attributing towards biohydrogenation :

- **For hand - fed ruminants,** the principal feeds, given in addition to leaves and stems (the so - called roughages), were cereal grains and these feeds comprised 2-5 % dry matter and in which 18:2 was the principal constituent.
- It was observed that the administration of oils per abomasums or duodenum, that is, by-passing the rumen, could markedly change the fatty acid composition of depot fat example, Palm or Rapeseed or Coconut oil containing polyun saturated fatty acids were infused into the proximal duodenum of rumen - fistulated and duodenal - T cannulated Holstein Friesian multparous cows. Calcium soap of Palm fatty acid - Megalac did not dissociate in the rumen, may be because, biohydrogenation could have been limited according to conjucture that **a free carboxyl group of the fatty acid molecule was pre–requisite for such reaction**.

It was opined that, as long–chain acids of dietary origin could be incorporated directly into the milk fat, the ratio of short and as long - chain fatty acids of as well as the degree of saturation of milk fat might be altered. The ability to alter the fatty acid profile of milk fat was limited not by the synthetic capacity of the udder, but rather by the challenge of achieving effective protection of unsaturated dietary fatty acids from biohydrogenation in the rumen, as well as keeping the level of PUFA **organoleptic quality** and **shelf - life** of milk and dairy products were not compromised. The fatty composition of oil seeds such as Palm or rapeseed were considered desirable from a human health perspective and thus, their inclusion in the diet of dairy cattle as a means of achieving a more desirable fatty acid profile in milk fat might enhance the nutritive quality of milk.

Avoid "Non-natural milk"

Feeding poly unsaturated fatty acids (PUFA) either protected or by-passed against ruminal biohydrogenation, would increase their proportion in milk, which would be a good answer to the guide - lines for human health. However, the most common treatments were either chemical (for example, Formaldehyde) or physical (for example, heating). The former would be difficultly /- accepted by consumers who wish to buy **"safe and healthy products"**; while the latter could enhance the proportion of *trans* isomers in the fatty acids and produce a **"non natural milk"**. Infact, fatty acids with *trans* isomers were usually considered to be related to sickness, for example, Cardiovascular diseases and Cancer. Therefore, it is important to increase the poly unsaturated fatty acids in the milk without increasing the proportion of their *trans* isomers.

- For grazing ruminants, the leaves and stems of grasses and forbes (especially clovers) provided the main source of feed. Lipids, chiefly in chloroplasts, usually comprised about 3 % dry matter, in which 18:3 was by far the dominant fatty acid.

- In tropical pasture plants, much lower 18:3 and much higher 18:2 proportions had been recorded.

These findings indicated that, while the lipids in ruminant diet tended to be highly unsaturated, the animal's depot fats tended to be highly saturated, which was due to biohydrogenation occurring in the rumen.

Lipid Metabolism in rumen

In an evolutionary sense, the rumen was developed as an expansion of the cardiac portion of the stomach. This milieu happened to be highly anaerobic and resulted in the production of hydrogen (10^{-4} atmosphere) and accounted for about 5 % of the total gases as a product of the binary - fermentation. The long chain unsaturated fatty acids were, therefore, hydrogenated, which were not further metabolized or absorbed in the rumen. As per another report, biohydrogenation occurred only after hydrolysis of the esterified fatty acids. Stearich acid was the end product of hydrogenation of linolelc and linolenic acids. It was observed in yet another study that some intermediates - *trans* **18 : 1** isomers, which resulted from the reduction of **18 : 2** and **18 : 3,** substantial part of both - structural and storage lipids in tissues and also of milk -fats. Although, microbial population contributed about 10-20 % of the lipids in the digesta (mainly branched chain fatty acids with 14, 15, 16 and 17 carbon atoms), but they had no 18 : 2 and 18 : 3 acids.

The capability of rumen microbes to hudrogenate unsaturated fatty acids were HIM demonstarated by R.Reiser in 1951. Thereafter, presence of PUFA was reported in the veal or lambs in the pre - ruminant state. Formaldehyde (now banned in U.S.A. !) treated oil -protein preparations were found to be protected *in vivo,* by feeding to lactating goats and cows. Encapsulated casein oil supplements were found to be entirely satisfactory for experimental use, were too expensive for commercial application. Therefore, the procedure was modified, so that natural oil seeds could be used as a source of both oil and protein. Thereafter, commercial scale -up plants were in operation in Australia, New Zealand and U.S.A. Some oil seeds, for example -Safflower had the advantage of higher proportion of 18 : 2, but the tough fibrous husks of commercial cultivars made comminution and emulsification more difficult; dehusking would avoid this difficulty, but oxidation of the kernels produced off- flavours in the milk products or meat, and also interfered with solubility characteristics of the oil seed globular proteins. Therefore, inclusion of an anti-oxidant, such as Ethoxyquin, solved these problems as well as solubility during storage.

Ruminants could tolerate a considerable level of dietary fat and as rumen being actively lypolytic. free fatty acids produced were not further degraded. Therefore, free fatty acids and fatty acid - soaps were **germicidal** and **bactcriostatic.** It was demonstrated that fatty acids inhibited methanogenic and cellulolytic species and Oleic acid was the most inhibitory of the series. Such inhibition was due to the **surfactant effect** of fatty acids which adhered to the bacterial cell walls and impeded the passage of essential nutrients. When the dietary lipid content was raised by the addition of unprotected fats, it was observed that a substantial fraction excreted in the faeces as soaps.

Chapter 29

Alkane Technology: An Extremely Powerful "User Friendly" Tool for Dairy Industry

Chemistry of Alkanes

In living plants, hydrocarbons are universally distributed in the waxy coatings on leaves and other plant organs. Alkane fraction is commonly a mixture of hydrocarbons of similar properties. The qualitative pattern is relatively similar from plant to plant, but there are considerable quantitative variation. Alkanes are saturated long chain hydrocarbons. They are usually present in the range of C_{23} to C_{33} carbon atoms. Examples are n-nonacosane, $C_{29} H_{60}$ and n-hentriacontane, $C_{31} C_{64}$. In general, odd-numbered carbon chains occur predominantly in the cuticular wax of plants and are substantially indigestible.

How alkanes are "user friendly" !

Following are some points to ponder :

- Alkanes are long carbon chains found naturally in plants and each plant species has its unique compliment of these different alkanes which act like **"fingerprints".** Forage intake can be estimated from 'faecal grab samples', if the ratio between these endogenous plant alkanes and exogenous alkanes delivered from **"a rumen slow - release gelatin capsule"** is calculated.
- Alkanes can also be used for determining digestibility and characterizing the species composition of the diet, making alkanes an extremely powerful tool for dairy research.
- An enexpensive, reliable and simple technique offers tremendous potential for research in the area of low cost dairy production from forages. Such data may be used by "slow–release marker" to estimate intake and digestibility.
- Alkanes offer a potentially simple technique for the animal scientist and it is feasible to estimate alkane concentrations using Near Infra-Red

scanning [N.I.R.]. It is a rapid analytical method, thus making alkane technology an extremely 'user friendly' tool to be widely adopted on behalf of the dairy industry.

What is creative here !!

Following dots would explain :

- The alkane slow - release marker estimates daily faecal output and digestibility of forages fed to cattle.
- Feeding level has no effect on digestibility estimated using the slow-release 'alkane marker'.
- Alkane concentrations in forages and faeces can be estimated by Near Infra Red reflectance.
- The alkane slow - release marker estimates the extract amount of each plant proportion of each plant species ingested in forage mixtures fed to **even female cattle**.

Why to choose such technology !!!

Following are the reasons

- A conventional digestibility trial is long, tedious, expensive and hence, a negative impact on the welfare of the animal (Un Ethical!).
- Animals have to be tied, all faeces must be collected and there must be no contact between urine and faeces to avoid contamination. As a result, it is very difficult to measure digestibility with dairy animals.
- Alkane markers offer a sound alternative. Additionally, they allow to assess intake of different plant species. This could help to improve pasture management by increasing our knowledge of animal's performance for plant species.
- Being of plant origin, alkanes are safe to use and milk does not have to be **with held**.
  - There are no health implications for the cows and this procedure could be used on farms to establish forage quality too.
  - It is critical to measure digestibility for avoiding nutritive value and dry matter in take of forages.

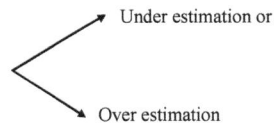

Chapter 30

Least Cost Accounting

For economical ration - preparation, selection of cheap feed among the locally available sources, is an important point to ponder. For this purpose, a list of available feeds is prepared alongwith their latest costs on dry matter basis. The cost per kg of dry matter is divided by the amount of the nutrient (as a decimal), it will give us a good idea of the :

- Cost of Crude Protein in → Protein supplements and,
- Cost of Energy in → Energy feeds.

For example, if alpha alpha hay costs Rs 3.93 per kg of dry matter, the cost per kg of Crude Protein = 3.93/0.171 = Rs 22.98 per kg.

In this way, it is possible to prepare a list of protein sources in the order of "Ranking" from which feeds can be selected at lower costs.

Effect of Differences in Dry Matter

Feeds are purchased on the basis of Dry Matter due to variation of moisture content. For example :

A Corn of 89 % Dry Matter costs Rs 7 per kg,

Another type of corn of 75 % Dry Matter can't be comparable on this cost This can be done as following :

0.75 / 0.89 XRs 7 = Rs 5.90

The underline cost guide for the selection of certain feeds for inclusion is a cost comparison of the primary nutrient to be provided. For example, a simplified comparison of Cotton seed meal to Soybean meal would be on the cost per unit of protein provided. If the computational data of the two feeds:

Commodity	Cost [say: dollar per pound]	CP %
Cotton seed meal (CSM)	4.20	41
Soybean meal (SBM)	4.95	45

[*Note:* Any unit of currency or weight can be used. Here, it is just an example].

Then, the cost per pound weight of crude protein would be 10.2 cents and 11.0 cents for CSM and SBM, respectively. Therefore, CSM is the more economical source of CP and, if all other nutrient aspects were comparable, would be the protein supplement of choice. However, there may be difference in energy value, mineral content and vitamin content, to say nothing of the fact that not all protein supplements give the response per unit of crude protein. Similarly, nutrient cost comparisons may be made on the other commodities.

Morrison in the year 1965 had tabulated data on the feed ingredients to calculate cost comparisons using Corn as the base energy feed and Soybean meal as the base protein feed. Comparative values using Barley grain and CSM have also been established. Such simplified procedures do not ensure that the final mixture will be the least possible cost, but **provide a rapid means of comparing cost.**

Linear Programming

It's a mathematical technique used for Least - cost ration formulation. These are handled easily by giving all the relevant details of different feeds including the costs to the "Computer-Memory". When the prices are changed, they are entered in the computer. Gradually, a data base gets prepared, hence such exercise guides us to chose the best feed among the lot.

Chapter 31

Abnormal or Fertilized Eggs of Hen should not be Marketed

Egg Formation Phenomenon

The chicken egg consists of a very small **Reproductive cell or Germinal disc [or Blastoderm;** which is capable of developing into an Embryo, if fertilized by a Sperm]. This tiny cell is surrounded by :

- Yolk

    = **OVARY** is responsible for its synthesis.

- Albumen, Shell membranes, Shell and Cuticle

    = These are produced in the **OVIDUCT.**

[A] OVARY

Although there are two ovaries and two oviducts in the hen, but only the left ovary and left oviduct are functional [because, the right ones are atrophied during embryo development]. Before egg production, the ovary is a group of small follicles of different sizes containing ova.

Formation of Yolk

- The yolk is just a source of food material for the small Reproductive cell (Blastoderm).
- Major amounts of yolk material is produced in the liver and transported to ovary through blood.
- Two days after the formation of First yolk. Second yolk begins to develop.
- It takes about ten days for a yolk to mature.

The colouring matter of the **Yolk**

Xanthophyll (a carotenoid pigment) is responsible for that characteristic orange-yellowish colour of the yolk. This pigment is derived from the feed, for example- Yellow corn.

[**Experiment:** Please check the colour of yolk in the broke - opened boiled egg. If it is any shade of dark or light orange - yellowish colour, yes, the farmer had fed his hens with good quality feed having plenty of Xanthophylls.

If the yolk colour is just white, then that farmer might **have cheated or what!!!**

Why we find alternate **rings of light and dark layers in the Yolk upon close examination!**

The flow of Xanthophyll is as following :

Feed (containing pigment) → **Blood** .... Quickly taken up by → **Yolk**.

- **During** day **time,** when the hens generally observed to be eating, there is uptake of Xanthophyll as shown in the above flow-sheet.
- **During nights,** when the hens observed to be not eating in general, there would be less accumulation of this pigment.

Hence, one can observe alternate rings of dark and light colour in the yolk. [Confirm under microscope]

OVULATION

At maturity, the ova are released from the ovary to enter the Oviduct. This process is called Ovulation and is initiated by both - Nervous and Hormonal systems. At this stage, **Yolk** membrane or **Vitelline membrane** is formed to hold the yolk contents together. The Second ovulation is regulated by the laying of the FIRST egg and it occurs 30 minutes after the First egg passes out through the cloaca.

[B] OVIDUCT

It is a long tube through which the yolk passes and where, the remaining portions of egg are secreted. Normally, it is relatively small in diameter, but with the approach of the FIRST ovulation, its size and wall thickness increases [as result of Follicle Stimulating Hormone (FSH)]. There are four segments of oviduct and are as following :

1. Infundibulum

It's a funnel shaped segment of the oviduct. When it is functional, its length is about 9 centimeters. Immediately after ovulation, its function is to search out and engulf the yolk and to cause it enter the oviduct. The yolk remains here for a brief period of 15 minutes and then forced along the oviduct by multiple contractions (wave like Peristaltic movements).

2. Magnum

This is the ALBUMEN (egg-white) secreting segment and is about 33 centimeters long in the average layer - hen. It takes about 3 hours for the developing egg to pass through the magnum. The albumen in an egg is composed of following 4 layers :

a) **Chalaza**
   [Chalazae is plural for two] = 2.7 % ⎫
b) **Inner white** = 17.3% ⎬ These first 3 layers are produced in the Magnum
c) **Dense white** = 57.0% ⎭
d) **Outer white** = 23.0 %   [But, this 4th layer is not completed here. Actually, water and salts are added in the Uterus for its completion].

Chalazae

These are two twisted cords extending from opposite poles of the yolk through the Albumen. These are produced due to twisting of yolk and therefore, chalazae are twisted in the opposite directions to **keep the yolk** centralized after the egg is laid.

Liquid Inner white

As the developing egg passes through the magnum, only one type of Albumen is produced, but the addition of water + rotation of the egg gives rise to various layers, one of which is the Liquid Inner white.

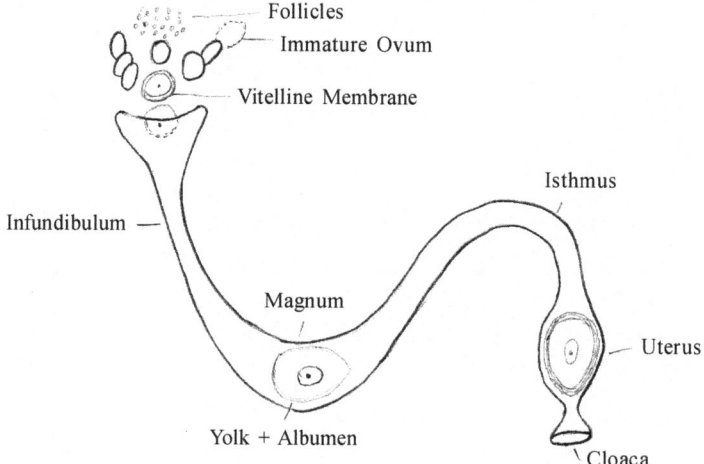

Fig. 6 : It is not normal to have 3 yolks in the oviduct at the same time. [This is just diagrammatic representation]

Dense white

The dense white makes up the largest portion of the egg albumen. It contains MUCIN, which tends to hold it together.

Outer white

This is completed in the UTERUS.

3. Isthmus

Now the developing egg is forced into the Isthmus, which is about 10 centimeters in length, where it remains for about 75 minutes. Here, the inner and outer shell membranes are formed in such a manner as to give the final shape of the egg. The shell membranes are a papery material, composed of protein fibres. The **Inner layer** is laid down first, followed by the Outer shell membrane, which is about 3 times thicker. Both the membranes are held closely together, but these two membranes separate to produce an "Air-Cell" at the large-end of the egg. The air-cell is about 1.8 centimeters in diameter. As the egg ages and interior contents dehydrate, the air cell increases in diameter and depth. The **size of air-cell is an indicator of the age of the** egg, because the contents continually dry out and the air cell becomes larger.

Functions of Shell membranes

a) They act as barrier to penetration by outside organisms, such as bacteria.

b) They also help to prevent the contents of the egg from evaporating rapidly and protect the egg contents.

4. Uterus

It is mainly the shell gland and is about 12 centimeters long in the layer - hen. The developing egg remains in the uterus for about 20 hours, much longer than any other segment.

a) **Formation of Outer Thin white :** This formed after the shell membranes are formed. This is the Magnum's incomplete layer, which is completed now. When the egg first enters the Uterus, water and salts are added through the shell membranes by the process of Osmosis to plump out the loosely adhered shell membranes and to liquefy some of the Thin Albumen to form the Fourth Layer, the Outer Thin white albumen.

b) **The Shell :** Small cluster of Calcium appear on the outer shell membranes just before the egg leaves the Isthmus. These are the initiation grains for Calcium deposition in the Uterus. There are two Shell layers :

i) **Inner Mammillary layer:** This is spongy and the first shell to be deposited over the initiation sites to form the inner shell. This is composed of Calcite crystals, which is sponge like material.

ii) **Outer Palisade layer:** The above layer is followed by the addition of the outer shell made up of a layer with hard Calcite crystals, chalky and about **twice thicker** than the inner shell surface. The longer the Pallisade columns, the stronger the shell. The completed egg shell is composed almost entirely of Calcite ($CaCO_3$), with small deposits of Na, K and Mg. On an average, there are 8000 pores in one egg shell. These are important for the exchange of Oxygen-Carbon Di Oxide and moisture for developing embryo.

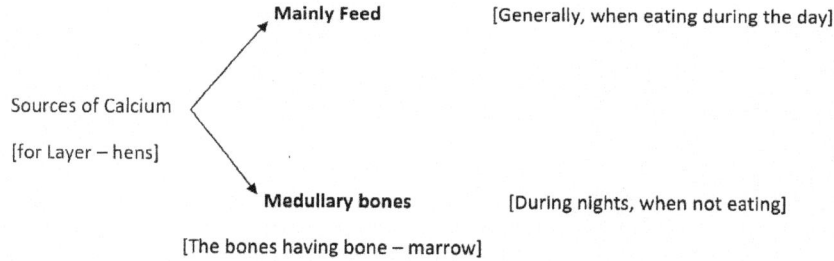

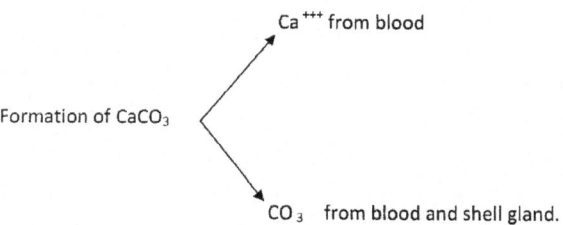

Calcium utilization

Requirement for Ca is extremely high. Calcium of total eggs produced per year per egg laying bird is 25 times more than the total calcium of egg laying poultry bird's skeleton. This is about 3-4 % of the ration per day. About 2 gms of Ca is used for each egg production in the laying hens.

Colour of the Egg - Shell

This may be white or various shades of brown. But, in South American chicken - the **ARAUCANA**, the eggs are of Green - Blue shells. The pigments responsible for shell colour are produced in the Uterus at the time of Shell formation.

Deterioration of Egg-Quality

After egg laying that is, OVIPOSITION, gradually there is constant change in the interior contents of the egg as following :

Egg-white (produced from Magnum)
  i) Dense white: the volume decreases and therefore becomes more viscous,
  ii) Outer white: the volume increases and therefore becomes more watery.

Air - Cell {produced from Isthmus)
Size of air cell increases.

c) The Cuticle

It is the last layer to be laid for egg - formation and is composed of Organic material. It acts as a lubricant during the egg - laying process. Later, it dries off.

CLOACA

It is the reservoir (like storage) for holding the completed egg. Throughout the oviduct, the egg moves small end first. But, just before laying, that is, OVIPOSITION, it rotates horizontally and large end of the egg is foremost. The rotation requires just 2 minutes. Such eggs are Infertile. They are called "Table Eggs" which are suitable for eating.

Fertilized Egg

If a male sperm comes to the funnel of the oviduct, penetrates the Vitelline membrane and joins the Yolk - Nucleus, this results in the production of "Fertilized Eggs". Such eggs are suitable for hatching purpose and therefore, also called as **"Hatching eggs"**. These eggs are not all used for table purpose.

ABNORMAL EGGS

1. **Double-Yolked eggs :** If two ova mature at the same time and enter into the infundibulum, such eggs are produced. This is because of over - active ovary during the initial stages of egg - Saying.

2. **Yolk-less eggs :** Stimulus produce by some blood clot or a piece of membrane in the oviduct and passing along in the same manner as the yolk, such eggs are resulted.

3. **An egg within an egg :** After an egg has been formed, it may be forced back upto the funnel region by reverse wave - like action. As it again

passes through the oviduct, the addition of Albumen, Shell - membranes and Shell are repeated and such eggs are produced.

4. **Foreign - matter in the egg** : Feather or any other substances fnd their way into the oviduct accidentially and become included in the albumen. They pass through the egg foration stages and become a part of the egg.

Appendices

Appendix 1: Nutrient Reqirements of Livestock
Daily Nutrient Requirements for Cattle and Buffaloes

Body wt. (kg)	Gain (g)	M.E. Mcal	C.P. (g)	Ca (g)	P (g)	Carotene (mg)
(1)	(2)	(3)	(4)	(5)	(6)	(7)
		Growing Animals (maintenance and growth)				
25	200	2.0	120	6	4	3
50	300	5.6	260	8	5	5
75	400	7.1	330	12	6	8
100	500	6.9	420(275)	16	8	11
150	500	9.1	565(245)	18	11	16
200	500	11.3	580(220)	20	13	21
250	500	13.4	680(200)	21	16	26
300	500	15.6	825(185)	23	17	32
350	500	17.9	985(180)	23	18	37
400	500	20.4	1170(185)	24	19	42

The figures in parentheses represent the requirements for Undegradable protein.

Maintenance of adult cows and buffaloes

Body wt. (kg)	M.E. Mcal	C.P. (g)	Ca (g)	P (g)	Carotene (mg)
300	9.7	290	14	7	30
350	10.9	325	15	9	36
400	12.0	360	16	11	42
450	13.1	400	18	13	48
500	14.2	425	20	14	53
550	15.2	460	22	16	58
600	16.3	490	24	17	64

Pregnancy allowance (add to maintenance) during last 2-3 months of pregnancy

Body wt. (kg)	M.E. (g)	Mcal C.P.	Ca (g)	P (g)	Carotene (mg)
1	2	3	4	5	6
300	2.8	280	8	6	16
350	3.2	290	9	7	19
400	3.5	300	10	8	22
450	3.7	310	12	10	25
500		4.0	320	13	1028

Milk Production (add to maintenance) per kg milk produced

Indian cow	1.4	100	2.9	2.2
Crossbred cow Jersey	1.4	100	3.0	2.3
Holstein Friesian	1.2	90	2.7	2.0
Buffaloes	1.8	120	3.4	2.5

Fat %		Based on Fat %		
3.0	1.0	64	2.5	1.8
4.0	1.2	80	2.7	2.0
5.0	1.4	95	2.9	2.2
6.0	1.6	105	3.1	2.4
7.0	1.7	120	3.3	2.6
8.0	1.9	130	3.5	2.8
9.0	2.1	140	3.7	3.0

For working bullocks

Body wt. (kg)	M.E. (Mcal)	C.P. (g)	Ca(g)	P(g)	Carotene (mg)
Moderate work (4h/d)					
300	11.1	460	10	10	16
400	14.4	575	13	13	21
500	17.3	680	15	15	24
600	20.1	760	17	17	27
Heavy work (8h/d)					
300	14.0	480	10	10	16
400	18.2	600	13	13	21
500	22.	730	15	15	24
600	25.8	850	17	17	27

Note
1. The figures for maintenance of cows and buffaloes may be used for idle bullocks.
2. For the maintenance of breeding bulls add 1.0 Mcal ME and 225g C.P. to the allowance for the same weight of cows.
3. When calculating the maintenance requirements for lactating first calvers that are still growing. The figures growth rather than maintenance should be used.
4. For cows producing more than 20kg milk per day. requirements are increased by 15 per cent.

Daily Nutrient Requirement of Sheep

Body wt.(kg)	Gain (or loss)	D.M.I. % of L.W.	M.E. or Metabolizable Energy (Mcal/Kg)	(Mcal/d)	Protein Total	DCP	Ca (g)	P (g)	Vitamin A (1000 IU)	Vitamin D (IU)

EWES AND LAMBS
Maintenance, Growth, Non-Lactating and First 15 Weeks of Gestation

10	50	3.9	1.95	0.76	35	18	2.3	1.5	1.9	64
15	50	3.5	2.00	1.04	49	25	2.8	1.8	2.9	196
20	50	3.3	2.00	1.29	59	31	3.3	2.3	4.0	128
25	100	3.3	2.40	2.00	85	48	4.2	2.8	5.0	164
30	125	3.1	2.75	2.57	103	60	4.9	3.3	6.3	199
35	125	3.1	2.75	2.89	177	69	5.9	3.3	4.1	218

EARLY WEANED LAMBS (5 to 30 kg)
Maintenance and Growth

5	100	2.3	4.3	0.50	45	36	1.8	1.3	0.50	35
10	100	2.1	4.0	0.84	70	56	2.1	1.5	0.85	67
15	150	2.3	3.8	1.30	109	87	2.7	1.9	1.28	98
20	150	2.3	3.5	1.61	135	108	3.2	2.2	1.70	133
25	200	2.5	3.1	1.91	160	128	4.1	2.8	2.12	168
30	300	3.3	3.0	2.95	248	198	5.0	3.3	2.55	200

Maintenance, Growth, Non-lactating and First 15 Weeks of Gestation

40	100	3.0	2.40	2.85	121	68	5.96	3.2	4.0	226
50	100	2.8	2.40	3.37	144	81	6.1	3.4	5.0	276
60	100	2.7	2.40	3.85	164	92	6.4	3.5	6.2	330

Daily Nutrient Requirement of Sheep

Body wt.(kg)	Gain (or loss)	D.M.I. % of L.W.	M.E. or Metabolizable Energy (Mcal/Kg) of diet	M.E. or Metabolizable Energy (Mcal/d)	Protein Total	Protein DCP	Ca (g)	P (g)	Vitamin A (1000 IU)	Vitamin D(IU)
Last 6 Weeks of Gestation or Last 8 Weeks of Lactation										
20	100	4.5	2.55	2.31	103	62	3.9	3.7	5.2	180
30	125	4.0	2.85	3.42	148	92	3.9	3.7	6.5	200
40	100	3.7	2.65	3.90	174	105	4.0	3.8	8.0	230
50	75	3.4	2.50	4.20	191	113	4.1	3.9	10.3	278
60	50	3.0	2.40	4.35	199	117	4.4	4.1	12.5	333
70	25	3.5	2.25	4.37	206	118	4.5	4.3	14.6	388
First 8 Weeks of Lactation										
20	5	5.0	2.35	2.34	105	60	9.5	6.9	5.9	180
30	5	4.5	2.20	2.99	143	82	9.8	7.1	6.8	200
40	10	4.2	2.00	3.37	176	101	10.4	7.4	8.2	235
50	20	3.9	2.00	3.99	209	120	10.9	7.8	10.3	278
60	30	3.8	2.00	4.57	239	137	11.5	8.2	12.5	333
70	30	3.6	2.00	5.13	267	154	12.0	8.6	14.6	388
RAMS Maintenance and Growth										
30	120	3.8	2.25	2.59	113	62	5.9	3.2	3.2	185
40	110	3.6	2.15	3.07	137	74	6.3	3.5	4.2	222
50	100	3.4	2.05	3.48	159	84	6.8	3.8	5.2	277
60	100	3.2	2.05	3.99	181	96	7.2	4.0	6.3	333
70	80	3.1	1.90	4.08	194	98	7.5	4.3	7.3	388
80	80	3.0	1.90	4.51	212	108	7.9	4.4	8.3	444
90	80	2.9	1.90	4.92	231	118	8.3	4.7	9.3	499

Daily Nutrient Requirement of Goat

Body wt.(kg)	Gain (or loss)	D.M.I. % of L.W.	M.E. or Metabolizable Energy (Mcal/Kg)	M.E. or Metabolizable Energy (Mcal/d)	Protein Total	Protein DCP	Ca (g)	P (g)	Vitamin A (1000 IU)	Vitamin D (IU)
5	25	4.4	2.35	0.52	22	15	0.8	0.6	0.4	78
10	50	3.7	2.50	0.92	39	26	1.5	1.2	0.6	139
15	50	3.3	2.30	1.13	48	33	1.9	1.4	0.8	169
20	75	3.1	2.40	1.49	63	43	2.4	1.9	1.1	232
25	75	3.1	2.30	1.67	71	48	2.7	2.1	1.2	247
30	75	2.8	2.20	1.84	78	53	3.1	2.3	1.3	273
40	100	2.5	2.30	2.34	99	67	3.8	2.9	1.7	353
50	100	2.4	2.20	2.62	111	75	4.3	3.3	1.9	395
60	125	2.3	2.25	3.17	134	91	5.0	3.8	2.2	465
70	125	2.2	2.15	3.35	142	96	5.5	4.1	2.4	507
80	150	2.1	2.20	3.75	159	108	6.3	4.7	2.7	573
Last 8 Weeks of Gestation and Last 8 Weeks of Lactation										
20	100	3.6	3.00	2.17	92	90	3.0	2.1	1.8	357
25	100	3.4	3.00	2.57	109	95	3.0	2.1	1.9	382
30	100	3.3	2.80	2.71	115	100	4.0	2.8	2.0	408
35	120	3.1	2.50	2.76	117	110	4.0	2.8	2.2	433
40	120	3.0	3.50	3.05	129	115	4.0	2.8	2.3	456
50	120	2.9	2.50	3.61	153	120	5.0	3.5	2.5	498
60	120	2.8	2.50	4.13	175	129	5.0	3.5	2.7	540
70	120	2.6	2.50	4.64	196	137	6.0	3.5	2.9	582

First 10 Weeks of Lactation									
20	-20	5.6	2.45	2.74	116	88	4.0	2.8	4.5	9.4
25	-20	5.4	2.30	3.02	128	97	4.0	2.8	4.6	929
30	-20	5.1	2.20	3.29	139	105	5.0	3.5	4.7	955
35	-20	4.9	2.10	3.54	150	113	5.0	3.5	4.9	980
40	-20	4.8	2.00	3.79	160	121	5.0	3.5	4.9	1003
50	-20	4.5	1.90	4.16	176	133	6.0	4.2	5.2	1045
60	-20	4.3	1.85	4.71	199	151	6.0	4.2	5.4	1087
70	-20	4.3	1.75	5.14	217	164	7.0	4.9	5.6	1129

Nutrient Constituents of Goats Milk at Different Fat Levels (Nutrients/kg Milk)

Fat (%)	Energy M.E. (Mcal)	Protein Total (g)	DCP	Ca(g)	P(g)	Vitamin-A (1000 IU)	Vitamin-D (IU)
2.5	1.20	62	42	2	1.4	3.8	760
3.0	1.21	66	45	2	1.4	3.8	760
3.5	1.23	71	48	2	1.4	3.8	760
4.5	1.26	79	54	3	2.1	3.8	760
5.0	1.28	84	57	3	2.1	3.8	760

Nutrient requirements, premix and ingredients for surine

Partculars Ingredients	Young Pre-Starter	Starter	Growing	Finisher	Pregnant sows/gilts	Farrowing/ lactating Sows/gilts
CP%	20	20	18	16	15	15
ME, Mcal/kg	3.35	3.35	3.17	3.17	3.15	3.15
Premix (kg/100kg)						
Salt	0.35	0.35	0.25	0.25	0.50	0.50
DCP	1.25	1.00	1.00	1.00	1.50	1.50
Limestone	0.50	0.75	0.75	0.75	0.75	0.75
Vit. mix.	0.10	0.10	0.075	0.05	0.10	0.10
Choline mix.	0.10	0.10	-	-	0.10	0.10
Biotin folic acid mix	-	-	-	-	0.05	0.05
Trace min. mix	0.10	0.10	0.075	0.05	0.10	0.10
Antibiotics (g)	10-25	10-25	5-10	05-10	-	5-15
Copper Sulphate	0.10	0.10	10-25 ppm	10-25 pmm	-	-
Total	2.5	2.5	2.15	2.10	3.10	3.10

Ingredients
1. Maize
2. Wheat
3. Barley
4. Rice polish
5. Soyabean meal
6. Fish meal
7. Meat cum bone meal
8. Ground nut cake
9. Fat

Note
A. For preparing meal mixtures for growing swine upto 30kg weight, following are added-
   a) 75% of basal feeds
   b) 15% Vegetable protein supplement
   c) 5.7% animal protein supplement
B. In case of swine having Between 30-50kg body weight, following are added-
   a) 85% of basal feeds   b) 9% Vegetable proteins
   c) 3% animal proteins

Nutrient Requirements For Poultry (per cent or in each kg of feed)

Nutrients	Broiler Starter (BSF)	Broiler Finisher (BSF)	Chick Feed	Growing Chicken (GCF)	Laying Chicken (LCF)	Breeder Chicken (BCF)
Metabolizable energy (Kcal/kg)	2900	3000	2700	2700	2700	2800
Protein (%)	22	19	22	16	18	18
Lysine (%)	0.9	0.9	1.0	0.7	0.5	0.5
Methionine (%)	0.35	0.35	0.35	0.25	0.25	0.25
Sulphur amino acid (%)	0.75	0.75	0.75	0.50	0.50	0.50
Linolenic acid (%)	1.0	1.0	1.0	1.0	1.0	1.0
Minerals						
Calcium (%)	1.0	1.0	1.0	1.0	2.75	2.75
Available phosphorus (%)	0.50	0.50	0.50	0.50	0.50	0.50
Manganese (mg)	60	55	55	55	55	55
Iodine (mg)	1	1	1	1	1	1
Iron (mg)	40	40	20	20	20	20
Copper (mg)	4	4	2	2	2	2
Zinc (mg)	50	50	-	-	-	-
Vitamins						
Vitamin A (IU)	6000	6000	4000	4000	8000	8000
Vitamin D (CD)	600	600	600	600	1200	1200
Thiamine (mg)	2	2	6	6	6	6
Riboflavin (mg)	5	5	5	5	5	5
Pantothenic acid (mg)	12	12	10	10	15	15
Nicotinic acid (mg)	40	40	30	20	20	20
Biotin (mg)	0.1	0.1	0.1	0.1	0.15	0.15
Vitamin B-12 (mg)	8	8	15	15	15	30
Alpha tocopherol (mg)	20	20	10	10	10	20
Cholin chloride (mg)	1400	1400	1300	-	-	1300
Crude fibre, (%) Max	6	6	7	8	8	8
Acid Insol, Ash, (%) Max.	3.0	3.0	4.0	4.0	4.0	4.0
Salt (as Nacl),(%) Max.	0.6	0.6	0.6	0.6	0.6	0.6

*CU stands for AOAC chick unit.

Appendices

Feed Requirements for Poultry (g)

Age in Weeks	Per Egg Laying Chicken		Per Broiler Chicken	
	Cumulative	Av. Daily	Cumulative	Av. Daily
01			84	12
02			294	30
03			609	45
04	650	35	1029	60
05			1554	75
06			2184	90
07			2919	105
08	1900	55	3759	110
12	3400	65		
16	5000	70		
20	7000	80		
24	10000	110		
30	14500			
40	22000			
60	37000			
80	52000			

Per cent Egg Production	Feed Requirement (g/bird)
0	80
20	90
40	100
60	110

Appendix-II: Nutritive value of common feeds (Straws and green forages)

Class of Forage	DM as Fed, %	Nutrient Composition on DM (%) basis					Voluntary Intake (kg DM/100kg)*
		C.P.	M.E. (Mcal/kg)	Calcium	Phosphours		
Straws and Karbies	90	3.0	1.6	0.15	0.08		1.5
Green sorghum, bajra, S.cane tops,							
Tropical grasses	25-40	6.0	2.0	0.50	0.30		2.0
Green maize	20-35	8.0	2.4	0.50	0.20		2.2
Green oat	20-35	10.0	2.4	0.40	0.30		2.2
Green berseem, Lucerne, Lobia	15-25	15-20	2.2	2.00	0.20		2.0**
		40			100		
		60			110		
		80			120		

*These figures are for desi cows and buffaloes. Crossbred cows eat about 25 per cent more than figures. Heifers of all breeds eat about 25 per cent more than adults.

**The consumption of Lucerne by buffaloes is only about 1.5 kg/100kg body weight.

Nutritive value of concentrate feeds on as fed basis

Feedstuff	D.M. %	Protein	Met. Energy (Mcal/kg) Poultry	Met. Energy (Mcal/kg) Cattle	Fibre %	Fat %	Ca %	P %	Lys. %	Methionine + Cystine %	Trypt. %
ENERGY FEEDS											
Cereal Grains											
High energy											
Bajra	90	10.8	2.61	2.55	1	5	0.12	0.4	0.39	0.18	0.20
Barley	90	10.1	2.69	2.80	6	2	0.08	0.2	0.58	0.38	0.19
Jowar	87	9.2	2.80	2.80	3	4	0.08	0.3	0.16	0.21	0.08
Maize	90	9.0	3.00	2.80	2	3	0.06	0.3	0.16	0.21	0.08
Wheat	90	11.5	2.70	2.80	2	2	0.06	0.4	0.42	0.42	0.17
Medium Energy											
Oat	92	9.5	2.68	2.68	11	5	0.10	0.3	0.38	0.39	0.18
Paddy	91	7.5	2.38	2.68	9	2	0.05	0.2	0.27	0.30	0.10
Roots											
High energy											
Tapioca chips	90	2.1	3.06	2.70	6	2	0.10	0.1	-	-	-
Factory by Product											
Feeds High energy											
Rice polish	92	11.0	3.13	3.00	4	13	0.10	1.0	0.40	0.28	0.08
Rice polish (Solvent extracted)	92	12.5	2.57	2.30	5	1	0.12	1.2	0.46	0.28	0.08
Medium energy											
Dal chune	90	13.5	1.1	2.2	12	4	0.40	0.3	-	-	-
Rice bran	90	12.1	2.64	2.35	12	11	0.16	0.9	0.50	0.30	0.10
Wheat bran	90	14.3	1.1	2.2	10	4	0.13	0.8	0.50	0.30	0.10
Low energy											

Feed										
Rice bran (solvent extracted)	90	13.1	2.0	2.0	13	1	0.17	1.0	0.58	0.35	0.12
PROTEIN FEEDS										
Vegetable Origin										
High protein										
Groundnut Cake	92	43.0	2.76	3.00	12	6	0.21	06	1.1	1.0	0.4
Deoiled GN Cake	93	47.0	2.50	2.66	10	10	0.23	0.6	1.2	1.3	0.5
Cottonseed Cake	92	27.9	1.66	2.58	20	5	0.48	0.8	1.0	0.9	0.4
Guar meal	90	36.0	-	2.16	12	8	0.48	0.6	1.3	0.4	-
Maize gluten meal	90	38.7	2.97	2.76	4	2	0.20	0.4	0.8	1.8	0.2
Sesame Cake	91	40.0	2.37	2.63	7	8	2.23	1.0	1.2	1.6	0.5
Deoiled Soyabean	90	48.0	2.83	2.99	5	1	0.32	0.8	2.3	1.2	0.5
Medium protein										
Mustard Cake	91	35.0	2.69	2.55	11	6	0.60	1.0	1.8	1.6	0.38
Linseed Cake	91	29.0	1.52	2.66	10	8	0.43	0.9	0.9	1.1	0.5
Low protein										
Coconut Cake	91	22.8	1.75	2.64	12	7	0.40	0.7	0.6	0.8	0.2
Maize gluten feed	92	22.8	1.70	2.66	8	2	0.44	0.8	0.8	0.6	0.2
Animal & Fish Origin										
High Protein										
Fish meal	94	56.0	2.73	2.71	-	7	7.00	2.8	5.9	1.85	0.5
Meat meal	92	45.0	2.54	2.56	-	9	7.48	3.9	3.7	1.35	-
Mineral Supplements										
Bone meal	96	11.5	0.55	0.55	-	3	25.8	11.0	-	-	-
Mineral mixture (Cattle)	-	-	-	-	-	-	28.0	12.0	-	-	-
Mineral Mixture (Poultry)	-	-	-	-	-	-	20.0	20.0	-	-	-
Shell grit	-	-	-	-	-	-	36.0	-	-	-	-

Miscellaneous									
Fat & Oils	98	-	7.5	4.5	-	98.0	-	-	-	-
Lucerne meal	91	17.0	1.35	2.04	25	2.5	1.3	0.60	0.8	0.5	0.4
Molasses	74	3.2	2.34	2.47	-	-	0.9	0.08	-	-	-

Source: All the tables of appendix I and II, Manohar Verma (1990); Prineiples of Animals Nutrition, Practical Exercise book; Earstwhile Animal Science, G.B.P.U.A.& T.; Pantnagar (Uttaranchal)

Some Important Books

Alkane Technology: Proceedings of the third International Symposium on the Nutrition of Herbivores (1991); Pennang, Malaysia (August 25-30; 1991).

An Introduction to Practical Biochemistry: Plummer, David T. (1979); Second edition; TMH.

Animal Feed Technology: Kundu, S.S.; Mahanta, S.K. Sultan Singh and Pathak, N.N. (2005); Satish Serial Publishing House, Delhi.

Animal Husbandry: Banerjee, G.C. (1999); Oxford and IBH Publishing Co. Ltd., New Delhi and Calcutta.

Animal Nutrition and Feeding practices: Ranjhan, S.K. (1998); Vikas Publishing House Pvt. Ltd.; New Delhi.

Animal Nutrition: Maynard Leonard, A. and Loosli John K., (1982); Sixth edition; TMH.

Animal Nutrition: Mc.Donald, P.; Edwards, R.A.; Greenhalgh, J.F.D. and Morgan, C.A. (1995); Fifth edition, Addison Wesley Longman, Inc., England.

Animal Nutriton in the Tropics: Ranjhan, S.K. (2004); Vikas Publishing House Pvt. Ltd.; New Delhi.

Basic Animal Nutrition and Feeding: Church, D.C. and Pond, W.G. (1982); John Wiley and Sons; New York and Toronto.

Biochemisrty: Lehninger, Albert L. (1978); Second edition, Kalyani Publishers (Indian edition).

Elements of Biochemistry: Gupta, P.K. (1999): First edition, Rastogi Publishers; Meerut.

Feeds and Principles of Animal Nutrition: Benerjee, G.C. (2000); Oxford and IBH Publishing Co. Pvt. Ltd.; New Delhi and Calcutta.

Hawk's Physiological Chemistry: Osier, Bernard A. (1971); Fourteenth edition; TMH.

Lignocellulose Biotechnology: Kuhad, R.C, and Singh, Ajit (2007); I.K.International Publishing house Pvt. Ltd.; New Delhi, Mumbai and Bengaluru.

Livestock Health and Management: Sharma, M.C. and Misra, R.R. (1987); Khanna Publishers, Delhi.

Nutrition and Dietetics under Clinico - Therapeutic Conditions of Pet and Farm Animals: Short Courses of Centre of Advanced Studies (March 20 - April 18; 2001), Animal Nutriton, Indian Veterinary Research Institute, Izatnagar, India.

Poultry Nutrition: Singh, K.S. and Panda, B. (1990): Kalyani Publishers; New Delhi.

Principles of Animal Nutrition and Feed Technology: Reddy, D.V. (2001); Oxford and IBH Publishing, New Delhi.

Principles of Animal Nutrition : Practical Exercise Book; Manohar Lal (1990); Earstwhile Animal Science Department, G.B.Pant University, Pantnagar; Uttaranchal (India).

Protection of Essential Fatty Acids from Biohydrogenation: Where are we now !!!

Raman Rao (2000): The Dissertation of Post-Doctoral Research submitted to "Dairy and Swine Research and Development Centre, Lennoxville (Quebec) JIM 1Z3; Canada".

Review of Physiological Chemistry: Harpar, Harold A.(1973); Fourteenth edition; Maruzen Asian Edition - The Kothari book depot, Bombay.

Text Book of Feed Processing Techniques: Pathak, N.N. (1997); Vikas Publishing house Pvt. Ltd.; New Delhi.

The Mineral Nutrition of Livestock: Underwood, EJ. and Suttle, N.F. (1999); CAB International, U.K.

Trace Elements in Human and Animal Nutrition: Underwood, EJ. (1971); Academic Press; Amsterdam, Boston, London, New York, Oxford, Paris, San Diego, Singapore, Sydney, Tokyo.

Zoo and Wild Animal Medicine: Murray E, Fowler (1986); W.B.Saunders Co., Philadelphia, London, Toronto, Mexico city, Rio de Janeiro, Sydney, Tokyo, Hongkong.

Question and Answer

Q.1 A farmer wants to prepare half quintal of concentrate mixture containing twenty percent protein for the livestocks. Oat (15% protein) & G.N.C. (40% protein) are available in the market. What option should be **tick marked (√)** in the following :
   a) 80 kgs of G.N.C. & 20 kgs of Oat ( )
   b) 80 kgs of Oat & 20 kgs of G.N.C. ( )
   c) 40 kgs G.N.C. & 10 kgs of oat ( )
   d) 40 kgs Oat & 10 kgs of G.N.C. ( )
   e) 40 kgs Oat & 60 kgs of G.N.C. ( )
   f) None of the above ( )

Q.2 If "Ash percentage" had been subtracted from hundred, what would be left ? **Tick mark (√)** your answer in the following :
   a) Nitrogen Free Extractive (N.F.E.) minus [C.P.%+C.F.%+E.E.%] ( )
   b) Inorganic matter ( )
   c) Organic matter ( )
   d) Moisture ( )
   e) None of the above ( )

Q.3 Heat regulation of animal body is regulated by these properties of water : (a) Very high heat conducting power (b) High specific heat (c) High dielectric constant (d) Highest latent heat of evaporation. **Tick mark (√)** your answer in the following :
   a) a,b,c are correct ( )
   b) a,b,d are correct ( )
   c) a,c,d are correct ( )
   d) b,c,d are correct ( )
   e) All of the above are correct ( )
   f) None of the above are correct ( )

Q.4 A farmer wishes to purchase a quintal of Maize grains. Two types of Maize grains -'X'&Y are available in the market at Rs.600/- & Rs.700/- per quintal, containing 20 % & 10 % moisture respectively. What option should be **tick marked** (√) in the brackets provided in the following :
  a) 'X' type with the total cost of Rs. 375.00 ( )
  b) Y type with the total cost of Rs. 375.00 ( )
  c) Y type with the total cost of Rs. 388.88 ( )
  d) 'X' type with the total cost of Rs. 750.00 ( )
  e) Y type with the total cost of Rs. 777.77 ( )
  f) None of the above ( )

Q.5 Total number of ATPs (Adenosine Triphosphates) produced after the complete oxidation of one molecule of Stearic acid (C_{18}) would be (answer in code only) :
  a) 134 b) 136
  c) 146 d) 148

  Tick mark (√) your answer in the following code :
  a) A,B,C are wrong
  b) A,B,D are wrong
  c) A,C,D are wrong
  d) B,C,D are wrong
  e) All of the above are wrong

Q.6 Time taken by the movement of egg formation from Ovulation to Oviposition is : (a) Twenty four hours (b) Twenty four hours & Thirty minutes, (c) Twenty four hours & Thirty two minutes. (d) Twenty four hours & Thirty four minutes.
  Select your answer from the codes given below :
  a) A,B,C are wrong   b) A,B,D are wrong
  c) A,C,D are wrong   d) B,C,D are wrong
  e) All are wrong

Q.7 In late seventies, Dagnela disease in buffalo was found to be linked with paddy straw feeding, which ultimately led to :
  a) Skin Dermatitis
  b) Disturbed eco-friendly feeding systems
  c) Selenium toxicity
  d) None of the above

Q.8 When a double - yolked hen egg (as observed in egg - candler) is hatched in the incubator - hatcher, then :
   a) Single chick is produced   b) Healthy twins are produced
   c) Weak twins are produced   d) No chick would be produced
   e) No conclusion can be drawn

Q.9 Founder of 'Science of Nutrition' was :
   a) Laplace   b) Babcock
   c) Lavoisier   d) Hopkins
   e) None of the above

Q.10 Suppose, the formation of the first Yolk (follicle) of a hen started on the first day of this month, which led into complete maturation. The fifth yolk would have matured on the following date of this month :
   a) 14   b) 15
   c) 16   d) 17
   e) None of the above.

Q.11 Name the Nutritionist (s), who had received **Nobel - Prize (Medicine)** for discovering a very important nutrient :
   a) Hart & Humphrey   b) Frederick Hopkins & Eijkman
   c) Stepp   d) McCollum & Davis.
   e) Hoist & Frolish

Q.12 Write 'T' for the true statement or 'F' for the false statement in the following. If the statement is false, underline the false part also :
   * Concentrates have more than eighteen per cent fibre.
   * Omasum provides additional storage space for the feed.
   * Protein supplements have less than twenty per cent protein.
   * Foreign bodies are retained in Crop of the poultry for longer periods.
   * Brewer's grains & yeasts are good sources for energy feeds.
   * Roughages have less than eighteen per cent fibre.
   * Reticulum squeezes out water from the feed.
   * Dinanath (Dinbandhu) is a good dry roughage.
   * Oligotrichs come under Rumen - Flora class.
   * Size of the rumen is eighty per cent of its body weight.
   * Yak is a non - ruminant.

* *Copra hircus* is sheep.
* Goat is a bovine.
* Mithun is a non - ruminant.
* *Ovis aries* is goat.
* Mohair is the product from sheep.
* Sus *domesticus* is a poultry bird.
* Camel is ruminant animal.
* Cat - gut is simple stomached pet animal.
* *Gallus domesticus* is swine.

Q.13 Fill in the blanks in the following :

* Lavoisier & Laplace had designed .... & by means of which, they demonstrated that.................. is the essential source of body heat.
* Dry roughages used for 'Storage purpose', are called ....
* Babcock conceived the idea of trying out rations made up entirely from .... for his experiment.
* Tallow is ....
* Crab-by prducts are the feed stuffs, classed as ....
* Succulent roughages used for 'Storage purpose', are called ....
* Belching in human being is analogus to .... in ruminants.
* Another name of 'Proximate analysis' of feeds is .... & it was devised by ....
* Lard is ....
* Vomitting in human beings is analogus to .... in ruminants.
* Normal rumen microflora in calf is established at an age of ....
* Lavoisier discovered that the .... was an .... process.
* On an average, an adult cow produces .... saliva each day.
* Cud is ....
* Nitrogen Free Exrtract (on fresh sample basis) - ....
• Vitamin A was discovered by ....
• .... Is the carbohydrate compound in the liver which combines with toxic chemicals and bacterial by-products for detoxification purpose.

- Metabolizable Energy minus Net Energy = ...
- Nutrient .... protects vital organs from mechanical shock and maintain body temperature.
- .... mineral is an extracellular cation.
- .... is the carbohydrate compound, which forms matrix of connective tissue.
- Gross Energy minus Metabolizable Energy = ...
- .... of lipids class, show hormonal activity in the animal body.
- .... is a mucopolysaccharide which acts as anti-coagualant.
- α .... is 25 % more biologically active form than to α ....
- Digestible Energy minus Metabolizable Energy = ...
- A carbohydrate substance .... is an important compound in tendon, cartilage, bone etc.
- .... mineral is an intracellular cation.
- .... of lipid class, acts as precursor of bile pigments, some hormones etc.
- Energy retention is also called as ....
- A carbohydrate compound .... is widely distributed in the plant kingdom and a number of them have been used as drugs for animals.
- Any two examples of essential amino acids are ....
- Deficiency of Vitamin K causes .... problem.
- Synthesis of bile acids, is the function of ....
- Chelate is a ....

Q.14 What was the conclusion of Hart & Humphrey's experiment about **"Something"** ?

Q.15 For which nutritional study, two experiments are conducted ? **Tick mark ($\sqrt{}$) yours answer in the following :**
   a) For Biological Value determination. ( )
   b) For indirect method of digestibility determination. ( )
   c) For Protein Replacement Value determination. ( )
   d) All of the above three - a,b,c are correct. ( )
   e) None of the above. ( )

Q.16 A cow had eaten 10 kgs of fresh Sorghum fodder containing twenty percent moisture and voided 1.5 kgs of dry matter in its faeces. Find the digestibility co-efficient of Sorghum. [Tick **mark** (√) yours answer in the following:

a) 0.25 ( )
b) 0.81 ( )
c) 25.00 per cent ( )
d) 81.25 per cent ( )
e) None of the above ( )

Q.17 Digestibility co-efficient for 'Ash' is not calculated, because :

a) It does not contribute energy. ( )
b) Pancreatic juice adds more minerals in the ash fraction. ( )
c) Bile juice adds more minerals in the ash fraction. ( )
d) All the above three - a, b, c are correct ( )
e) None of the above. ( )

Q.18 Which Vitamin has the following function? Write answer in space provided.

a) As a biological anti-oxidant......................
b) Protecting epithelial tissues and mucous membrane ....
c) Helping in ElectronTransport Chain ....
d) Helping in Oxidation-Reduction reactions ....
e) Helping in the activity of Parathyroid hormone ....
f) In combination of Se, prevents Encephalomalacia ....

Q.19 Name the type of category, the minerals carry out their following function

a) For maintaining acid-base balance in the body ....
b) For binding with some enzyme ....
c) Bonding of Iron in the Cytochromes ....
d) Bonding of Iodine in the Thyroxine ....
e) Bonding with other minerals in the bones ....
f) For maintaining osmotic pressure in the body ....

Q.20 Deficiency of which Vitamin or mineral causes following problem in farm animals.

a) Pica
b) Muscular dystrophy
c) Milk fever
d) Fatal sycope

Q.21 Write the formulae for the following :
   a) Total Digestible Nutrients %
   b) Protein Efficiency Ratio
   c) Starch Equivalent
   d) Protein Replacement Value
   e) Digestible Crude Protein % of maize fodder
   f) Biological Value.

Q.22 Briefly give reasons for the following :
   a) In the indirect method of determining digestibility, what "assumption" is made ?
   b) Lipid delays hunger.
   c) Approaches for 'Protein evaluation' is different in ruminant and non-ruminant ?
   d) It is said that protein and fat are burnt in the flame of carbohydrate.
   e) Lipid is the most concentrated form of stored energy,
   f) Calves don't have rumen.
   g) Fibrous feeds serve as "Rumen-fill".
   h) Foreign bodies are retained for longer periods in one of the stomach compartments
   i) Why is it called 'Crude' in :
      i] Crude Protein
      ii] Crude Fat

Q.23 Draw diagram of poultry alimentary canal.

Answer

Note:

1. Answers have been given in the descending (reverse) order of question-numbering.
2. For some answers, we have to look in the referred chapters of this book.
3. We should not always ask Google or Wikipedia for information. Afterall, our whole life is a "do it yourself project".

23. Please refer to Figure 2 of chapter 4.

22. Reasoning questions:
    a) It would be **"assumed"** that the digestibility coefficient of nutrients in the roughages obtained from the First trial would remain the same in the Second trial, where concentrates are mixed with this roughage. Therefore, the total nutrients voided in the faeces from the portion belonging to roughage in the First trial is subtracted from the Second trial to get the remaining nutrients belonging to Concentrates, which would be considered to have come from the concentrate-feed being tested.
    b) This is because; **lipids require longer time** to pass through the stomach than carbohydrate or protein.
    c) In the simple stomached animals (including we humans), the proteins containing polypeptides are broken down to oligopeptides, which are further broken down to amino acids. And then, these amino acids are assimilated or utilized. In ruminants, all the above degradations are also going on. But, here, **even the amino acids are also broken down.** And secondly, **synthesis of new proteins also takes place by microbes for the synthesis of their own body coat proteins.** Because of these reasons, the approach for protein evaluation is different.
    d) Certain intermediary compounds of Glucose oxidation through Kreb cycle are absolutely necessary for oxidation of proteins and fats.
    e) Because lipids provide 2.25 times per unit more energy than carbohydrate.
    f) Calves have **Reticular or Oesophageal groove (a tube)** in place of Rumen and its continuation Reticulum. This tube directly opens into Abomasum (that is, the true stomach).
    g) Fibrous feeds are bulky. The Crude Fibre is **Hydrophilic** (that is, water loving) and hence swells, leading to 'Rumen fill'. Moreover, passage of digesta is also slow.

h) Reticulum provides additional space plus 'Foreign bodies' like - nails, wires etcetera, which are retained for longer periods, to prevent damage of soft organs.

i) Crude Protein = In addition to 'True Protein', they have Non Protein Nitrogen (NPN) compounds, for example - Urea, amino acids, amines, amides, nitrates, purines, pyrimidines, some 'B' complex Vitamins, some N - containing lipids etcetera. Crude Fat = While extraction of sample with Petroleum Ether, some Organic acids, Organic alcohols. Plant pigments also get mixed alongwith lipids in the fraction due to solubility.

21. For the formulae, we have to refer the Chapters-6 and 8 of this book.

20. The deficiency of following nutrients are responsible for such problems
    a) Phosphorous deficiency in cattle.
    b) Vitamin E deficiency in cattle.
    c) Calcium deficiency in dairy cow.
    d) Vitamin E deficiency in Swine.

19. Following are the function-type of mineral
    a) Electrochemical function (for example, Na, K, Cl)
    b) Catalytic function (for example, Mg)
    c) Chelating function (for example, Fe in Cytochrome)
    d) As a constituent (for example, Iodine in Thyroxine)
    e) Structural function (for example, Ca and P in bones)
    f) Electrochemical function (as above).

18. (a) E; (b) A; (c) K; (d) C; (e) D; (f) E.

17. d (all the above - a,b,c are correct).

16. d

15. d (all of the above three - a,b,c are correct).

14. Either, Wheat plant contained 'Something',

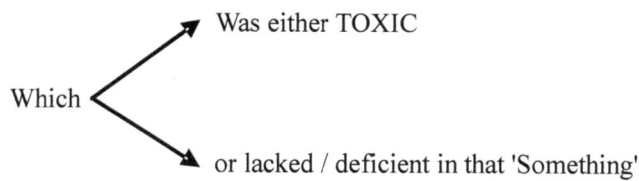

Or, that 'Something' was **supplied by the Corn plant.**

At that time, they could not name that 'Something'.

[It was years later that the new discoveries provided the true answer.

13. Fill in the blanks:
    - Calorimeter, respiration.
    - Hay
    - Single plant
    - Cattle fat
    - Protein supplement
    - Silge
    - Eructation
    - Proximate analysis; Hanneberg ane Stohman
    - Swine fat
    - Regurgitation
    - Six weeks
    - Combustion, Oxidation
    - 100 to 200 litres
    - Half digested feed
    - N.F.E. [Fresh] = C.P.% + E.E. % + C.F. % + Ash % + **Moisture %**
    - Me Collum and Margurette Davis (1913).
    - Glucuronic acid
    - Heat Increment
    - Lipid
    - Sodium
    - Hyal Uronic acid
    - Digestible Energy
    - Prostaglandins
    - Heparin
    - Tocopherol; Tocotrienol
    - Urinary Energy + Methane Energy
    - Chondroitin sulphate
    - Potassium

Question and Answer 207

- Cholesterol
- Net Energy for production
- Glycosides
- Essential Amino acids-Arginine, Histidine, Isoleucine, Leucine, Lysine, Methyl Alanine, Phenylalanine, Threonine, Tryptophan, Valine.
- NIL [because, this vitamin is synthesized by ruminants as well as plant feeds have plenty of this vitamin].
- Lipid
- In Greek language, Chelate means **Claw.** It is a Cyclic compound formed between an Organic Molecule and a Metallic ion.

12. All are **false.** Now we can underline the false parts.

11. b

10. Say, if the First Yolk formation started on April, 01st, then formation of 5th Yolk would begin on April, 19. [Because of the following as per the literature survey:
    - Two days after the formation of First Yolk, Second Yolk begins to develop.
    - It takes 10 days for a Yolk to mature.
    - April 1, 3, 5, 7, 9 + 10 days = April 19].

9. c (Lavoisier).

8. d (no chick would be produced, because that was abnormal egg).

7. c (Selenium toxicity).

6. b [that is, 24 hrs and 32 minutes].

5. c [(5 ATPs produced per β Oxidation cycle x 8 β Oxidation cycles = **40 ATPs) plus** (12 ATPs per Acetyl Co A produced in Kreb cycle x Total of 9 Acetyl Co A molecules = **108 ATPs) minus** 2 ATPs expended during initial activation of fatty acid) = 146].

4. d ['X' type with total cost of Rs. 750 /-].

3. b (a,b,d are correct, refer to this book).

2. c (Organic matter).

1. d (40 kgs of oat and 10 kgs of GNC).

Index

A

Abnormal Eggs 178
Albino 39, 40
Allowance 43, 45, 70
Antelopes 107
Ants 107
Aquatic types 107
ARAUCANA 177
Arboreal 107
Argentation chromatography 181
Ass 113
Atrophied 173
Attrition mill 91
Aureomycin 11, 75

B

Bamboo 108
Banyan 6
Barley 7, 8, 9, 36, 73, 95, 117, 172
Beans 7, 9, 10, 103
Bean 9
Biotin 60, 89, 137
Blastoderm 173
Blood meal 10
Bovimax 137
Bran 2, 8, 68, 73
Buffers 11, 13
Butylated hydroxyl toluene 11

C

Camel xii, 114, 115, 186
Carnivore 105, 106, 108, 111
Casein xi, 11, 39, 59, 60, 101, 104, 167
Chalaza 175
Chevon 37
Chicken 31, 37, 104, 112, 125, 173, 177
Choline 10, 60, 72
Chromatoaraphy 165
Clover 6, 7, 30, 39, 115
Coffee 6
Colostrum 60, 69, 70, 71, 72
Corn cobs 7
Cotton 3, 6, 7, 89, 93, 126, 139, 171
Covit 137
Crumbles 93, 98, 148

D

Data Base 107, 172
Deer 107, 115
Dental care 104
Dental pad 86
Dermatitis 184
Digestibility 2, 3, 10, 33, 34, 35, 37, 38, 40, 41, 56, 71, 94, 108, 117, 119, 120, 169, 170, 187, 188, 189, 190
Dog Chow Cheker 103
Double Pearson Square 139
Draff 9
Dystokia 68

E

Elephant 111, 112, 113
Eructation 29, 32, 192
EUN 40
Extrusion 92, 94
Fatal sycope 188
Feather meal 10, 94
Feedex 137
Felids 111, 112
Fish meal 3, 10, 55, 94
Folic acid 102
Formula 40, 49, 69, 98, 99, 105
Fossorial 107
Founder of science of nutrition xi

G

Gazelles 107
Gelatinization 94
Germinal disc 173
Growth waves 53, 54
Guillotine ix
Guinea pigs 41

H

Hammer mill 90, 91
Hazsard Analysis and Critical Control Point (HACCP) 150, 163
Herbivores 112, 115
Hippopotamus 108, 114
Hippopotamus 108, 114
Horn buttons 76
Horse 9, 48, 90, 109, 113, 114
Huempe 117

I

Immunoscreening 121
Impala 107
Infundibulum 86, 174, 175, 178
Inositol 60
Isthmus 176, 178

K

Kapok 6, 126
Kernel 2, 3, 8, 95, 126
Kitten 105, 106
Kjeldahl's method 39
Kudus 107

L

Ligninase 120, 121, 122, 123
Linear Programming 154, 155, 156, 157, 172
Lucerne (alpha alpha) 7

M

Magnum 175, 176, 178
Maize 7, 89, 10, 33, 34, 62, 103, 184, 189
Mammillary layer 177

Mastication 29, 31, 38, 85
Mastitis 68, 77
Meat meal 10, 94
Melanin 15
Methane 32, 37, 38, 48, 192
MFN 40
Micronizing 95
Middling 2, 104 136
Milk fever 68, 188
Muscular dystrophy 188
Mutton 37

N

Neutraceuticals 104
Nicotinamide 10
Non-protein 10, 39, 48

O

Oat 3, 7, 8, 34, 103, 115, 139, 142, 183, 193
Orphans 105
OVIPOSITION 178, 184
Ovulation 174, 184

P

Paddy 7, 71, 117, 126, 127, 184
Pail 72, 73
Peas 7, 9, 103
Pebble mill 146
Peepal 6
Pelleting 90, 92, 93, 143, 148
Penicillin 11
PICA 188
Pinnipeds 111
Piperazine 78
Polypropylene 102, 119
Popping 95
Pork 37, 89
Poultry xii, 3, 8, 9, 10, 34, 37, 39, 45, 57, 83, 90, 98, 104, 112, 126, 127, 182, 185, 186, 189
Prehension 29, 85
Premix 133, 134, 135, 136, 137
Prills 63
Protected-fat 63
Pseudo-ruminant 114
Pyridoxine 126

R

Rabbits 39, 50, 112
Rennet 11
Rhinoceros 108, 113
Rhodopsin 15
Riboflavin 8, 9, 10, 11, 60, 72
Ringing 84
Rod mill 145
Rumen-fill 34, 189
Rye 7

S

Safety factor 43, 44
Salivation 29, 31
Silages 7
Single cell protein 10
Skim milk 11, 72, 73, 84
Slivers 8
Solid not fat 11
Sorbitol 101
Spectroscopy 165
Spent hops 9
Suckling 29, 69, 88
Surfactant 168

T

Tape shooter 98
Taurine 106
Terrestrial 107
Territorial 114
Tetracycline 11
Thiamine 60, 72
Thyroxine 15, 188, 191
Total digestible nutrients 5, 35, 189
Trimming 84

U

Udder 59, 60, 61, 63, 64, 67, 68, 69, 72, 81, 88, 166
Uterus 175, 176, 177

W

Weaning 1, 69, 71, 72, 75, 106
Wheat 3, 7, 8, 36, 73, 74, 104, 117, 119, 126, 136, 147, 191
Wistar rats 39

X & Z

Xanthophyll 173, 174
Zebra 113

CPSIA information can be obtained
at www.ICGtesting.com
Printed in the USA
BVHW091131240223
659163BV00015B/1022